AF352539

# GLOBAL HEALTH AND THE VILLAGE

Transnational Contexts Governing
Birth in Northern Uganda

SARAH RUDRUM

# Global Health and the Village

## Transnational Contexts Governing Birth in Northern Uganda

UNIVERSITY OF TORONTO PRESS

Toronto  Buffalo  London

© University of Toronto Press 2022
Toronto Buffalo London
utorontopress.com

ISBN 978-1-4875-0455-7 (cloth)    ISBN 978-1-4875-3043-3 (EPUB)
ISBN 978-1-4875-3042-6 (PDF)

---

**Library and Archives Canada Cataloguing in Publication**

Title: Global health and the village : transnational contexts governing birth in
    northern Uganda / Sarah Rudrum.
Names: Rudrum, Sarah, author.
Description: Includes bibliographical references and index.
Identifiers: Canadiana (print) 20210291761 | Canadiana (ebook) 20210291907
    | ISBN 9781487504557 (cloth) | ISBN 9781487530433 (EPUB) |
ISBN 9781487530426 (PDF)
Subjects: LCSH: Maternal health services – Uganda – Amuru District. | LCSH:

    Childbirth – Uganda – Amuru District. | LCSH: Medical assistance – Uganda
    – Amuru District. | LCSH: War and society – Uganda – Amuru District. |
    LCSH: Public health – International cooperation. | LCSH: World health.
Classification: LCC RG966.U332 A48 2022 | DDC 362.1982/0096761 – dc23

---

This book has been published with the help of a grant from the Federation
for the Humanities and Social Sciences, through the Awards to Scholarly
Publications Program, using funds provided by the Social Sciences and
Humanities Research Council of Canada.

University of Toronto Press acknowledges the financial assistance to its
publishing program of the Canada Council for the Arts and the Ontario Arts
Council, an agency of the Government of Ontario.

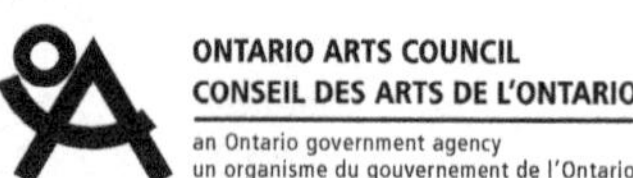


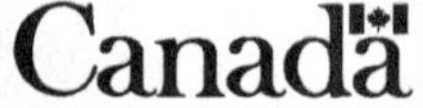

# Contents

# Acknowledgments

It is a pleasure to be sharing this work. I am able to do so because of help along the way.

In Uganda, health workers and researchers lent their enthusiasm and expertise to this project. Many staff members at Lacor Hospital and Lacor Health Centre III welcomed us warmly, as did those at St. Anthony of Padua parish and school. I am of course particularly indebted to the mothers and health workers who participated in interviews and focus groups. *Apwoyo matek.*

I am grateful to the two anonymous reviewers who offered sound advice and insights, and to the staff at University of Toronto Press for guiding the way. My colleagues and friends at the University of British Columbia and at Acadia University offered support and were part of many conversations that have helped shape this work.

Thank you to the readers who will keep this conversation going.

I would also like to acknowledge the scholarships and awards that have helped fund my work in Uganda. Thanks to the University of British Columbia for doctoral funding, to UBC's Liu Institute for Global Issues for fieldwork support, and to the Harrison McCain foundation for a research award I received at Acadia University.

I'm grateful to my parents, June and Alan, and my sister, Katy, whose pride, interest, and encouragement have been invaluable. Omar Bhimji and Sachaa Rudrum-Bhimji, you have shared the journey, including any detours and roadblocks. Many thanks and much love to all of you.

⌇⌇⌇

Ethics approval: At the University of British Columbia, the Behavioural Research Ethics Board approved the research proposal. It was titled

"Women's Approaches to Childbirth in Northern Uganda." The certificate number is H11–02573. Within Uganda, this project received ethics approval via the Lacor Hospital Ethics Review Board, the Uganda National Council for Science and Technology, and the Office of the President (file number SS 2846).

# Acronyms and Abbreviations

| | |
|---|---|
| ANC | antenatal care |
| DHO | district health officer |
| HIV | human immunodeficiency virus |
| HSM | Holy Spirit Movement |
| IC | Invisible Children |
| IDP | internally displaced people |
| LC I | local councilperson (level I) |
| LRA | Lord's Resistance Army |
| MDG | Millennium Development Goal |
| NGO | non-governmental organization |
| NLA | National Liberation Army |
| NUMAT | Northern Uganda Malaria Aids and Tuberculosis Project |
| SBA | skilled birth attendant |
| TBA | traditional birth attendant |
| UMOH | Uganda Ministry of Health |
| UNAIDS | The Joint United Nations Program on HIV/AIDS |
| UNFPA | United Nations Population Fund |
| UPDF | Uganda People's Defence Force |
| VHT | village health team |
| WHO | World Health Organization |

# Glossary of Terms

*apwoyo matek*   thank you very much
*boda-boda* **(or simply** *boda***)**   motorcycle taxi
*cen*   a spirit or an apparition, usually evil; a polluting spiritual force
*mandazi*   fried bread
*mic*   a gift
*ot yat*   hospital or health centre
*panga*   machete
*pii oo*   waters burst
*pime*   measurement
*posho*   pancakes
*Plumpy'nut*   a brand of peanut-based paste used to treat malnutrition
*raah*   grass
*Rwot Kweri/Rwodi Kweri*   traditional leader(s)
*simsim*   sesame seeds
*waragi*   a strong clear alcohol

GLOBAL HEALTH AND THE VILLAGE

Transnational Contexts Governing
Birth in Northern Uganda

# Chapter One

# Introduction to a Crisis in Maternal Health

## Introduction

For those who work in maternal health, the word *preventable* is a source of deep frustration alongside persistent optimism. The knowledge that most maternal deaths could be avoided through basic and well-understood measures makes the high numbers of women dying globally in childbirth not only tragic but also senseless and vexing, as with the inequities in the geographic distribution of such deaths. While countries such as my own, Canada, have succeeded in bringing maternal deaths down to an irreducible minimum, in many countries, rates remain high. Uganda is one such country.

In a setting of mounting frustration and anger as maternal deaths in the country continued unabated, a recent legal struggle drew attention to the dire state of maternity health care in the country and attempted to catalyze change. Irene Nanteza died of haemorrhage following a ruptured uterus; the doctor on duty had failed to report to work, arriving hours after the initial crisis, at which point it was too late for medical intervention (Center for Health, Human Rights and Development [CEHURD], 2012). The constitutional challenge alleged that the Ugandan government had violated the human rights of Nanteza and another woman, both of whom died while giving birth in state hospitals. The claim was that "non-provision of essential maternal health commodities in government health facilities, leading to the death of some expectant mothers, is an infringement on the right to health of the victims" (CEHURD, 2012).

Spearheaded by CEHURD, this landmark case was the first to test the government's legal obligation to provide care to birthing women. In 2015, four years after Irene Nanteza's death, the High Court found in favour of CEHURD and Nanteza's family, awarding damages. A lack of supplies and the absence of skilled staff were found to have contributed to these preventable deaths.

Inadequate investment in facilities, staff, and equipment can lead to care that is best described as "too little, too late" for parturient women who reach a health facility (Miller et al., 2016). Many other women, among the approximately 58 per cent who give birth without a formally trained attendant,[1] die alone or in family settings. Pregnancy is relatively frequent in Uganda, with an average of 6.8 children born to each rural woman in 2011, dropping to 5.9 by 2016 (Uganda Bureau of Statistics, 2011, 2016). The deaths brought forward by the CEHURD case speak to the maternal health challenge in Uganda. An important indicator of the relative safety of pregnancy and birth in a given setting is the maternal mortality ratio, which tracks maternal deaths per 100,000 live births, recording deaths in childbirth and those that occur because of pregnancy-related causes during or soon after pregnancy. The maternal mortality ratio is "an internationally accepted marker of the safety or otherwise of pregnancy" (O'Hare & Southall, 2007, p. 565). In 2011, Uganda's maternal mortality ratio was calculated at 438 per 100,000 (Uganda Bureau of Statistics, 2011); expressed another way, this meant about 6000 women were dying each year (Sebina-Zziwa et al., 2013). More recently, this ratio has dropped to 336 per 100,000 – still among the highest maternal mortality ratios in the world (Uganda Bureau of Statistics, 2016). Pregnancy and birth remain unnecessarily dangerous for women in Uganda and elsewhere on the continent.

In 2012, I moved with my family to a rural northern Uganda health centre located at a former internal displacement camp. The majority of people in the north had been relocated to such camps during the protracted conflict between the Lord's Resistance Army and government forces that took place between 1986 and 2006. Living among my Acholi neighbours as they rebuilt their homes, farms, and lives post-conflict, I set out to understand how maternity care and childbirth were organized in this remote agrarian region of northern Uganda recovering after decades of armed conflict. In the process, I not only gained a detailed understanding of the particular challenges Acholi women in Amuru faced in accessing safe maternity care services but also learned

---

1 In sub-Saharan Africa, approximately 58 per cent of women delivered their first child outside a health facility (Rogo, 2006). Many of these births are attended by a traditional birth attendant (TBA). In Uganda, Grace Kyomuhendo's study in a rural area of western Uganda also found that 58 per cent of women gave birth outside a health facility (Kyomuhendo, 2003). Poor women throughout the region are more likely to give birth at home (Montagu et al., 2011).

how these were shaped by shortcomings in how the problem of maternal mortality is approached by global health organizations. As well as focusing on local cultural, social, economic, and health system factors shaping maternity care and birth, my research thus extended to an analysis of the encounter between ambitious and standardized global health goals and the local realities of a remote post-conflict community with poor health services.

I came to understand that global health goals and policies were successful in their scope, in that they impacted care even in this remote community, yet failed in particular ways to meet local needs. As necessitated by resource constraints and a mismatch between available supports and local needs, international health interventions were reinterpreted in the national and local context, a practice Julie Livingston has referred to, in the Botswana context, as "improvising care" (2012). These insights on improvised care can be extrapolated to the post-conflict health care context in northern Uganda. Muyinda and Mugisha (2015) draw on the concept to suggest that "while improvisation is a feature of biomedicine and facilitates problem solving in daily life," the context of post-conflict health care delivery necessitates better and more strategic global north–global south collaboration on more equal terms so that health workers aren't simply being called on to use "less effective or non-recommended procedures" (p. 316). Improvisation is necessary in health care, but when it becomes a major characteristic of how health care is delivered, it can signal failure to supply the necessary basics for providing care. Interrogating how culture and technical problems are framed in international health interventions, it becomes clear that the objectifying and colonizing premises on which interventions are often based means that rather than being "unanticipated," the negative consequences that too often result from international interventions in health are structurally determined. *Global Health and the Village: Transnational Contexts Governing Birth in Northern Uganda* examines this interplay between localized social relations and transnational politics as they organize maternity care and birth.

Guiding my research was the following question: *How are maternity care and childbirth socially organized in the context of Amuru sub-county, a rural area recovering from conflict in northern Uganda?* My focus on social organization was deliberately broad to enable me to account for the numerous overlapping factors that might influence care and birth. Family settings, community settings, and health care settings all feature in the organization of maternity care and birth, while factors including access to resources, geographic location, and cultural practices are each likely to exert their influence. In the face of a trend towards uniformity and standardization, there is a counter appeal in which many scholars have called for context-specific research and practice in global maternal health (Kyomuhendo, 2003; MacKian, 2008; Say & Raine, 2007; Spangler, 2011; Sundby, 2014). My detailed focus on a particular geographic and social context in this research responds to that call. Starting from this specific context, my view of the social relations around maternity care grew to encompass transnational global health relations. The goal was to understand the local birthing and maternity care context, beginning with the experience and standpoint of birthing women using institutional ethnography (IE) approaches. I mapped the social coordination of maternity care and birth in Amuru sub-county, starting with the accounts of birthing women and going on to interview health workers and administrators. To supplement these interviews, I turned to analyses of texts, discourses, and policy documents related to maternity care. Maternity care and childbirth are important areas of inquiry and intervention throughout sub-Saharan Africa, a region in which maternal mortality is the highest in the world; this research began from the standpoint of birthing women in this particular Acholi community in northern Uganda.

## Contexts of Care

### Health Care Provision

In Uganda, health services are decentralized and are identified by levels corresponding to local political entities. A health centre (HC) I corresponds to the village level; it has no physical facility and solely comprises village health team (VHT) members, laypeople who receive some training and supplies and volunteer to be the first point of contact between individuals and the health care system (Uganda Ministry of Health [UMOH], 2010, p. 9). An HCII is the lowest level of health centre to have a physical facility. An HCII corresponds to the parish level so that each parish should have an HCII, though not every parish does. An HCII is designated to treat common illnesses and dispense drugs; the most senior staff person required is an enrolled nurse. An HCIII, like Lacor HCIII where I lived, corresponds to the sub-county level. The most senior staff member required is a senior clinical officer, and HCIIIs are also required to have the capacity for blood transfusions and emergency surgeries, as well as a lab and a lab technician. An HCIV is required to have a doctor and an operating theatre, in addition to the staffing and facilities of lower-level centres, and serves a county. The highest level of care is offered at hospitals, which should be able to offer specialized services in each district, with complex cases referred to regional and national referral hospitals (Institute for Health Metrics and Evaluation [IHME], 2014). There is a mix of public, private, and non-governmental organization (NGO) health care provision at all levels above the VHT (with VHT training also supported publicly and via various NGOs and religious groups). Within Uganda, because of staffing and funding shortages, not all health centres are able to function to their designated capabilities, as I saw in Amuru (Munabi-Babigumira et al., 2019). Relatedly, not all jurisdictions have their designated health centre, although overall physical infrastructure is more available than human resources, equipment, and supplies (Munabi-Babigumira et al., 2019). UMOH (2006) acknowledges such gaps, reporting that despite requirements, "most HCIIIs have no water and lighting for the maternity units while most HCIVs lack functional operating theatres and have inadequately skilled medical officers, unable to perform EmOC [emergency obstetrical care] and newborn care tasks yet a primary objective of establishing HCIVs was to provide facilities for comprehensive EmOC services such as caesarean sections and blood transfusion" (p. 11). Such gaps between the vision for the health care system and its reality affect all areas of care, including maternity care services.

*Background on the Millennium Development Goals (MDGs)*

Understanding maternity care in Amuru meant attention to major international policies and practices governing global health alongside localized practices at the health centre or in the villages. Among macro-scale global health practices, the Millennium Development Goals (MDGs) loomed largest. These eight goals for international development were adopted by world leaders at the United Nations in 2000 to be achieved by 2015. Upon their expiry, they were superseded by the Sustainable Development Goals (SDGs), and because they were active at the time of the research discussed, I focus here on the MDGs. MDG 5 was "to improve maternal health" and had two targets, 5.A, "reduce by three quarters the maternal mortality ratio," and 5.B, "achieve universal access to reproductive health." Target 5.B of the goal was a controversial late addition (in 2005) and was less prioritized than 5.A, which can therefore be understood as the substantive priority in improving maternal health (Yamin & Boulanger, 2013). This lack of a broader focus on sexual and reproductive health has been a point of critique of the MDGs, which undid previous international cooperation towards a sexual and reproductive rights agenda (Yamin & Boulanger, 2013). Those championing women's rights have argued that greater foregrounding of gender and rights would have improved results for the MDGs. As well as being reliant on other sexual and reproductive health rights, maternal health is inextricably connected to health issues addressed in other goals, particularly MDG 4 on reducing child mortality and MDG 6 on combating HIV, malaria, and other diseases. However, there was a lack of coordination in programs designed to address each goal. Progress on reducing maternal mortality was measured by two indicators: the maternal mortality ratio itself and "the proportion of deliveries attended by skilled health personnel" (World Health Organization [WHO], n.d.).

The MDGs have been criticized as "imprecise and ineffective" (Attaran, 2005, p. 0955) and as a "global wish list" (Saith, 2006, p. 1168), critiques similar to those now being made about the SDGs (Abe et al., 2015; Horton, 2014). Progress on MDG 5 on maternal health was noted to be difficult to measure because of lack of reliable data, particularly because "it is exactly in the poorest countries where the maternal mortality problem is severest that the data about deaths and births are least satisfactory" (Attaran, 2005, p. 0958). An additional problem was that the language of the MDGs was deliberately simple and streamlined to facilitate clear communication, but when the goals were shifted to national planning contexts, their generality made them "entirely inappropriate" (Yamin & Boulanger, 2013, p. 75). The MDGs use in policy planning was an extension of their scope and was particularly relied on by aid-dependent countries (Yamin & Boulanger, 2013), such as Uganda. For example, Uganda created a roadmap for reducing maternal mortality and morbidity that stated, "The overall goal is to accelerate the reduction of maternal and neonatal morbidity and mortality in Uganda and help the country achieve the MDGs" (UMOH, 2006, p. 7). As the deadline approached, it became clear that the goal would not be met: a 2013 report identified Uganda's progress on MDG 5 as stagnant and predicted that Uganda was "unlikely to meet the targeted reduction in maternal mortality" by the deadline (Uganda Ministry of Finance, Planning and Economic Development, 2013, p. 24), which it indeed did not. Internationally, MDG 5 made the least progress and was the least adequately funded of the eight goals (Barros et al., 2010, p. 1877; Women Deliver, 2009). Despite these criticisms and failures, MDG 5 was the clearest articulation of an international goal on maternal health and an international approach to maternity care provision. It was an important influence on how target countries, such as Uganda, approached maternal health and maternity health care, and it shaped both local and transnational approaches to maternal health.

In response to global health bodies advocating for broad goals on maternal health, many authors have called for more context-specific research into maternity care and birth in low-income countries in the global south[2] (Kyomuhendo, 2003; MacKian, 2008; Say & Raine, 2007; Spangler, 2011). Subtle and complex individual-level factors, such as perceptions regarding formal care and preference for the social support of traditional care, shape the unequal use of maternal health care (Say & Raine, 2007). Local perceptions regarding birth and care need to be understood and considered for interventions at the level of health services to have a significant impact (Say & Raine, 2007). While reducing maternal mortality through promoting the increased use of skilled attendants at birth has been identified as a goal across global contexts, understandings rooted in specific places and among specific people are necessary to make progress towards reducing maternal mortality (Say & Raine, 2007). In her discussion of inequality and social exclusion as they affect childbirth in Tanzania, Spangler (2011) makes the case that "to be effective, services must explicitly meet the needs of societies' most marginalized – they must ensure equitable access in unique contexts" (p. 493). As did these authors, I came to understand that standardized approaches to the maternal health problem, however laudable on their face, create problems when context-specific social factors are poorly understood or are overlooked.

### Skilled Birth Attendants (SBAs) and Traditional Birth Attendants (TBAs)

It is commonplace to distinguish between skilled birth attendants (SBAs), who have formal medical training, and traditional birth attendants (TBAs), with current policy approaches favouring the former. The term *TBA* is used by policy actors, NGOs, and scholars across national contexts to describe women who provide maternity health care but are not formally credentialed, although the practices, roles, and skills of TBAs vary within and between national contexts. One Ugandan researcher defines a TBA as follows:

---

2 I occasionally use the terms *global south* and *global north* to point to the features this study's setting shares with other parts of sub-Saharan Africa and with low-income countries on other continents, and to contrast the setting not only to Canada but also to other countries with similar economic profiles. Unlike the term *developing countries*, *global south* does not indicate that these countries need to catch up to "developed countries." While the term *global south* is preferable to *developing countries*, it is not ideal. In using it, I do not intend to disregard the tremendous in-country disparities of health, income, and status in global north countries such as Canada or to suggest that countries within the global south are more similar than different.

a person recognized by her community as able to assist women in childbirth. These practitioners are the "*mothers of the village*" because they assist in reproductive health care, like family planning, birthing, prevention of sexually transmitted HIV/AIDS counseling, promotion of immunization and breastfeeding. (Kyomugisha, 2008, p. 11)

However, such a broad and positive definition of TBAs would be perceived by many as out of step with efforts to limit the role of TBAs in favour of SBAs.

An important context for maternity health care in Uganda is the widespread but contentious use of TBAs. Relying on TBAs for labour support is widely viewed as problematic because it is seen as antithetical to the development goal of promoting reliance on SBAs, which has been identified as the primary means of reducing maternal mortality (Achadi et al., 2012; Say & Raine, 2007; Wirth et al., 2008; WHO, 2014). This is exemplified by the prominence of "proportion of births being attended by skilled health personnel" as an indicator for measuring progress on the reduction of maternal mortality in the MDGs. Globally, a widespread focus on training TBAs as a means to reduce the incidence of maternal mortality began in the 1970s, but scepticism about this approach emerged in the subsequent decades (Van Lerberghe & De Brouwere, 2000). The WHO, for example, promoted the training of TBAs between the 1970s and 1990s but has not since (Harrison, 2011; Sibley et al., 2009). Within Uganda, a ban on TBAs as sole attendants at birth has been discussed, and even announced, but never legislated. Reading the local papers, I observed a prominent idea that women's "shunning" of formal care contributes to maternal mortality.[3]

Despite the scrutiny surrounding the use of TBAs by birthing women in Uganda and elsewhere, the issues contributing to the prevalence of birth at home with TBAs are not fully understood. A 2003 review of maternal health in Uganda conceded that

> the overall status of women, social expectations to deliver at home, and demands on women's time have all been identified as factors leading to

---

3 For example, headlines include "Pregnant Women Shun Hospitals" (Ahimbisibwe, 2004); "Kaberaido Mothers Shun Hospitals" (Nauele, 2010); "Why K'jong Women Still Shun the Labour Ward" (Emasu, 2006); "Pallisa Mothers Shun Antenatal Care" (Kolyangha, 2011). Kyomugisha (2008) quotes an MP as stating, "Despite the government's efforts to bring health services nearer to the people, some women still die with maternity complications because they don't use the health centre services ... 30% of women die every year because they have shunned the use of modern medical facilities and prefer to use the traditional methods, which put their lives at a great risk" (p. 20).

home delivery and use of TBAs rather than trained medical birth attendants for delivery assistance. However, there are clearly also technical access barriers (such as geographical distance from facilities or cost) which may prevent utilisation of services, and issues with the quality of care available in facilities. It is important to disentangle the web of access barriers to identify the way these various factors are interrelated. TBAs may be socially more appropriate for some women, but they may also be particularly preferred when there is a perception of low quality in public health centres. Similarly, transportation barriers exist, but other factors may increase the delays in seeking care, thereby making early planning to offset transportation barriers more difficult. (Ssengooba et al., 2003, p. 29)

This excerpt elucidates the complexity of factors influencing women's practices regarding care during birth. It further suggests that "barriers to access" and "cultural preference" cannot be understood or addressed as separate factors shaping care. Instead, they are interrelated in context-specific ways such that learning from birthing women is key to understanding the interplay between technical barriers that limit access and social factors that shape preferences. A narrow focus on provider preference and barriers to skilled attendance may obscure attention to other everyday material contexts affecting care. Questions surrounding women's choices regarding care and barriers to accessing health care, despite signalling important topics, too often stall at blaming lack of patient demand (women's choices) or at narrow technical questions on barriers, overlooking the broader social, political, and economic landscape in a given context.

SBAs are defined as those with formal medical training (Campbell & Graham, 2006; Say & Raine, 2007). However, the definition of *formal training* ranges from describing any medically trained attendant as an SBA (Say & Raine, 2007) to the relatively narrow definition of "midwives and doctors" (Campbell & Graham, 2006, p. 1292). For example, the WHO (2004) defines an SBA as someone "trained to proficiency in the skills necessary to manage normal deliveries and diagnose, manage or refer obstetric complications," (pp. 3–4) but Harvey et al. (2004) assert that the "WHO's estimates [on attendance by a SBA] implicitly assume that anyone categorized as health personnel qualifies as a skilled attendant" (p. 204). In Uganda, policies promoting skilled attendance at birth have been hampered by recruitment challenges, hindering health facility capacity (Munabi-Babigumira et al., 2019). While TBAs have skills that are recognized by their communities, their lack of formal education excludes them from the category of SBAs. This is stated explicitly for the Uganda context: "TBAs are not considered skilled attendants at birth, even if trained" (Republic of Uganda, 2008, p. 48). Despite this, some authors have made the case for the continued importance of TBAs in improving maternal health outcomes based on factors such as preference and the ability of TBAs to work in hard-to-reach communities (Ana, 2011; Jokhio et al., 2005, Ray & Salihu, 2004). For example, Turinawe et al. (2016) argue that policy bans against TBAs are overly medicalized and neglect social context, and are thereby likely to "reproduce the inequities in health that they seek to address" (p. 10).

Alongside a focus on skilled attendants, the related concept of "skilled *attendance*" emphasizes that, in addition to the presence of those with midwifery skills, an "enabling environment" is required to support safe birth (WHO, United Nations Population Fund [UNFPA], 2014). Such an environment provides the resources required to deliver care, including "facilities, supplies, transport and professionals to provide emergency obstetric care when it is needed" (UNFPA, 2014, p. 2). Skilled attendance facilitates safe birth, but it is difficult to provide or access in many contexts, often including low-resource, rural areas. The controversy around TBAs' role is important to how childbirth is organized in the communities where they practise, including Amuru sub-county.

**Social Contexts for Maternity Care and Childbirth**

A focus on local contexts of care and birth means paying attention to social relations. When it comes to access to care, there can be a tension between the policy environment and social contexts. This is evidenced in the tension between the lack of accessible care available to women in Uganda and the discourse outlined above of women "shunning" formal maternity care. A similar tension emerges in Sara MacKian's (2008) research on representations of women's health in Ugandan newspapers, in which she found that "although the current policy climate aims to encourage women to utilise formal health provision, they are often the least able to negotiate access effectively" (p. 112). MacKian suggests that a supportive community-level environment may be key to negotiating care. There is a need to better understand how "women's participation might be encouraged beyond the more obvious routes of providing services and attempting to 'educate' them to change their ways" (p. 112). Dominant discourses, such as the need to provide health education, powerfully shape women's health and health care in Uganda. Grace Kyomuhendo (2003) characterizes the national context of maternity health care as one in which improvements have been made to policy but not to practice. While it was once justifiable to blame maternal mortality and morbidity on poverty and instability, she argues that this is no longer the case because of "good policies on gender equity, universal primary education, reproductive health and decentralisation of health services" (2003, p. 17). (This assessment is focused on a region that has been politically stable for some time, unlike northern Uganda, which faces ongoing instability in the aftermath of decades of conflict.) Specifically, the favourable policy environment has not been met by an increase in the number of women seeking formal care or by reduced rates of maternal mortality (Kyomuhendo 2003). Kyomuhendo attributes this to a "lack of resources at all levels, from facilities and staff to drugs and blood" (2003, p. 17) yet takes cultural beliefs regarding pregnancy as a central focus:

> The clinical causes of maternal deaths, the characteristics of women who die and the causes inherent to the health care system are well known in Uganda and elsewhere. Less is known about the cultural beliefs that may contribute to women's deaths. Many authors believe that maternal mortality in Africa has been influenced by socio-cultural beliefs, including gender and power relations, and differences in roles and status between the sexes. (p. 17)

Kyomuhendo identifies a dearth of literature on the sociocultural aspects of maternity care in Uganda and a need for attention to sociocultural factors influencing birthing experience and maternity care. However, as maternal mortality frames the concern with sociocultural aspects, the work links cultural beliefs to death in a way that places blame with women and culture for health concerns that are also shaped by sociopolitical factors, including structural violence.

Two major factors stand out as shaping health during pregnancy and birth in Kyomuhendo's (2003) study of birth in western Uganda: the first is a belief that birth is "a thorny road," inherently difficult and dangerous, and a woman's burden to bear; the second is birthing women's negative accounts of nurse-midwives as bossy, rude, and hurried. Some women felt that hospital staff "ignored the value and meaning they attached to their birthing experiences" (pp. 21–22) while health workers often viewed birthing women as ignorant or as having overly high expectations, oblivious to health workers' time and resource constraints.

Birth practices can also be connected to beliefs about gender and power. For example, among the Banyoro, "one who experiences no problems and needs no assistance is held in much esteem, having walked bravely through the hazardous path and emerged unscathed" (Kyomuhendo, 2009, p. 231). This perspective is seen as contributing to the limited uptake of skilled attendance. However, Kyomuhendo also acknowledges that cultural diversity within Uganda means such observations are not broadly applicable. In a study of "near-miss" experiences, this balance between social and health system factors is summarized as follows:

> Severe maternal illness is not necessarily a result of direct (biomedical) causes *per se* but may stem from other factors deeply rooted in culture and gender relationships. These factors notwithstanding, women are hampered by deficiencies in the formal health care system including *inter alia* inexperienced health workers, especially at lower level units, poor referral systems and the lack of a well-functioning transport system, limited space in the wards or operating theatre, and inability to access the busy health staff. (Kyomuhendo, 2004, p. 1)

A similarly wide-ranging set of factors was identified in a study located at a public sector health facility in northern Uganda, where negative provider-patient interaction, poverty, and health system deficiencies were noted as factors impeding health centre delivery among women who did attend antenatal care (ANC) (Anastasi et al., 2015). While social factors affect how health care is accessed, ultimately an inadequate health system means that understanding health provision contexts remains essential to understanding women's approaches to care.

*The Post-conflict Setting*

The health centre in Amuru was at the site of a former internal displacement camp. Some remnants of the camp, such as broken standpipes and partial walls, still dotted the property. Families were in the process of returning home and rebuilding their huts and family gardens. Agriculture was the primary way of life and economic activity in this rural community, and most Acholi are Christian. These contexts, as well as the conflict and post-conflict context, are discussed in greater detail in chapter 2.

The decades-long conflict between the Lord's Resistance Army (LRA) and Government of Uganda forces, and the concomitant mass displacement of the majority of civilians, remains a major social force during the post-conflict and return period, which I explore in chapter 2. Amuru sub-county is in the process of recovery and rebuilding after the end to the conflict in Uganda's northern region through a ceasefire agreement signed in 2006 between the LRA and Government of Uganda forces. Since the end of armed conflict, or indeed during those years, there has been little study of maternity health care and childbirth among the

Acholi people. However, what is known makes clear the need for further research focusing on maternity health care and childbirth experience with an understanding of the post-conflict setting in this region.

With regard to conflict settings more generally, maternal mortality is significantly higher in sub-Saharan African countries that have recently experienced conflict than in those that have not (O'Hare & Southall, 2007, p. 565). In broad terms, we know that conflict is detrimental to maternal health: "a complex humanitarian emergency imposed on an already weak health system compounds the risk of maternal death" (Austin et al., 2008, p. 914). However, the specific points of weakness affecting childbirth and maternity care in the context of post-conflict northern Uganda are poorly understood. A study of perceptions of the effects of the armed conflict on maternal health among stakeholders in Burundi and northern Uganda found that worry over increased morbidity and mortality was paired with an acknowledgment that social consequences of war, such as increased prostitution, had consequences for maternal health (Chi et al., 2015a). An interesting feature of post-conflict in this region is that it can, perhaps surprisingly, mean less access to care for many civilians than they had during the conflict itself. Conditions during displacement were overall poor, but formal care provision was present in the camps, via health centres, in a way that it had not been otherwise for many residents. This meant that, in the north, the overall rates of skilled assistance were actually higher during some years of the conflict than in the rest of the country where peace prevailed (Namasivayam et al., 2017). Since returning to their homes, many women now live further from care, contributing to the difficulty of access. On the health provision side, providing access to safe care is constrained by human resources challenges in rural post-conflict northern Uganda: it is difficult to recruit specialists, including midwives, leading to staffing shortages that can result in burnout and, particularly at government-run centres, absenteeism (Chi et al., 2015b). The challenges I discuss regarding ANC care are also demonstrated in analysis of demographic survey statistics from the post-conflict period (Namasivayam et al., 2017).

## Methodology and Methods

*Key Institutional Ethnography Definitions:*
*Institutions, Participants, and Work*

This work relies on institutional ethnography (IE), an approach to social research developed by Canadian sociologist Dorothy Smith. Research in the IE tradition investigates processes of social organization by learning about people's everyday actions and experiences and how they are coordinated via institutional processes. Smith's insights leading to the development of IE were grounded in the Canadian women's movement as she worked to bridge the gap between women's lived social realities as mothers and sociological and institutional paradigms of motherhood (Griffith & Smith, 1987; Smith, 1987, 1997).

Since these first feminist inquiries, the IE tradition has fostered social change scholarship in various areas, prominently including health research in North American contexts (Mykhalovskiy & McCoy, 2002; Rankin, 2015; Sinding, 2010). Little IE research focuses on global south or transnational settings, although the few exceptions (Campbell & Teghtsoonian, 2010; Grace, 2013, 2015; Jakubec & Campbell 2003) show its potential. While global health scholarship has not typically taken up IE methodologies, after studying institutional ethnography with Dorothy Smith, I recognized that, for an inquiry centring women's experiences of and perspectives on health care that took into consideration their social setting and the health care setting, IE was the best fit. IE lends itself to context-specific research on health care as it was designed to explore how everyday activities in a given setting relate to forms of social organization extra-local to that setting. For researchers, "actual practice – how things actually work – becomes the focus of investigation" (Grahame, 1998, p. 352).

As Eric Mykhalovskiy and Liza McCoy (2002) suggest, IE's focus on "how people's daily lives and troubles are organized socially and institutionally" (p. 20) is conducive to the creation of knowledge supporting equity, representation, and inclusion, especially in the setting of political struggles. An IE approach to methodology, then, is epistemologically consistent with a conceptual approach guided by social justice. Christina Sinding (2010) identifies that "IE studies begin ... by drawing forward the activities, knowledge, and concerns of a group of people related to their involvement with a particular institutional complex" (p. 1657). In this way, I worked with IE methodologies to draw forward the activities, knowledge, and concerns of childbearing women in relation to the institutional complex organizing maternity care and childbirth. Attention to childbirth and maternity care in this setting was relevant not only because of poor outcomes but also because appropriate care and support is intrinsically important to women's lives, health, and well-being. My point of entry was the concerns of childbearing women; my research scope moved up and out from there. This orientation, in tandem with my extensive fieldwork period while based at a former internal displacement camp in this rural, post-conflict setting, helped to anchor the study in the context-specific social and discursive constitution of maternity care and childbirth. The potential of ethnography to address complexity in health research by investigating relationships and their unexpected results has been acknowledged (Huby et al., 2007); IE has been particularly useful in exploring these complex dynamics. Specific features of IE that were relevant to this work include approaches to institutions, participants, work, texts, and discourse. Each is briefly outlined below.

INSTITUTIONS

*Institutions* within IE are broadly defined to acknowledge how institutional influences are pervasive beyond the "walls" or formal bounds of self-described institutions, such as a hospital (Mykhalovskiy & McCoy, 2002). Key to the understanding of institutions within IE is a focus on what actually happens in day-to-day practice. Within IE, an *institution* refers "to a complex of ruling relations – the multiple activities of individuals, organizations, professional associations, agencies and the discourses they produce and circulate – that are organized around a particular function such as healthcare or education" (Mykhalovskiy & McCoy, 2002, p. 19). It is these activities and discourses I considered as I worked to understand the social organization of maternity care and birth in Amuru.

PARTICIPANTS AS EXPERTS

Research participants are not considered to be the objects of study in the IE approach, but rather expert informants on their own experiences as they intersect with the wider social phenomenon that is being researched. In such an approach, presenting people's assessments of health care delivery can be a form of advocacy, as it offers an orientation "toward the organization of health service delivery (what is being evaluated) and prevents it from stalling at a typology of evaluative criteria (studying the patients)" (McCoy, 2006, p. 117). Creating a typology is something for social justice researchers to avoid; centring the expertise of participants is one way to avoid objectifying and colonizing practices. Research that objectifies or others the participants can lead to findings that are judgmental, either blaming participants or casting them as victims with little agency. This is captured by Chandra Mohanty's transformative "Under Western Eyes" (1988), in which she argues that Western feminist discourse has constructed the category "third world woman" as homogenous, powerless, and victimized (p. 338). This over-determined view can mean that the specific material realities of specific women or groups of women are overlooked (Kumar, 2013; Mohanty, p. 338). Approaching participants as experts rather than as the objects of study decentres the researcher's role as expert and can contribute to social justice research practices.

## WORK

IE uses a broad definition of "work" as a way to understand the organization and significance of people's ordinary activities; it is not limited to paid employment. Work is "intentional: it is done in some actual place under definite conditions and with definite resources, and it takes time" (Smith, 2005, p. 154). Mykhalovskiy and McCoy's (2002) use of the concept "health work" to help understand the work that people living with HIV/AIDS undertake in managing their health exemplifies this approach. "Health work" included "the wide range of practices that people engage in around their health, without defining in advance what that work might or should involve" (p. 24) and took place within the larger institutional complex of health care. Other studies of health care in developed countries have interpreted the activities patients undertake in adhering to treatment routines, or seeking medical care more generally, as "work" (Lowndes, 2012; Sevigny, 2012). Attention to work and health work is particularly apt in a setting such as rural northern Uganda, where access to the basic amenities for coordinating health care – transportation, communication technology, and money – is so scarce. By paying attention to the work participants did in relation to maternity care and birth, I learned of work that took place in relation to health care provision, such as planning for transportation, and work that took place in relation to family and community, such as smearing the hut (resurfacing the floor). Further, I learned that certain approaches to HIV testing and to NGO programming introduced work for childbearing women that might have been unanticipated by policymakers. Understanding this work through an IE lens allowed me to expand and, at times, refocus my mapping of the social organization of maternity care and birth.

## TEXTS

Texts, broadly defined as written or graphic materials that can be reproduced and are used in coordinating translocal activities, are key in an IE approach. Texts produced in one place are influential in coordinating activities and knowledge in a different place and so act as an important bridge between local contexts and broader, or extra-local, contexts:

> The magical character of replicable texts from the point of view of institutional ethnographic interest is that they are read, seen, heard, watched in particular local and observable settings while at the same time hooking up an individual's consciousness into relations that are translocal. (Smith, 2006, p. 66)

To understand this coordination between local and extra-local contexts, institutional ethnographers pay attention to when texts are consulted or invoked.

An additional consideration regarding texts was how the contexts of low literacy and low media consumption influenced the circulation and operationalizing of texts, a consideration I explored in an article on the need to adapt IE methodologies for use in global south contexts (Rudrum, 2016a). Scholars of IE have often situated the importance of texts in historical contexts that are particular to the industrialized global north, in contrast to a rural setting in the global south. For example, Dorothy Smith (2002) situates her discussion of texts in European history and North American politics, concluding her study of how texts facilitate ruling relations by stating, "Advanced contemporary industrialized societies are pervasively organized by textually mediated forms of ruling" (p. 212). Campbell and Gregor (2002) refer to how *literate* people put texts into action in everyday life (p. 32), while Smith (2006) labels texts as "those most commonplace objects of our contemporary world, so much present that we take their ubiquity entirely for granted" (p. 26). Daniel Grace (2013) asserts that "in late (post) modernity institutional knowledge is text-mediated" (p. 38). These examples demonstrate that the cultural shifts making texts so central to organizing knowledge and activities have not occurred universally; these scholars do not theorize the role of texts in societies that are not characterized by industrialization or the ubiquity of media. Therefore, while previous IE writing on texts was influential, it was necessary for me to think through how texts worked within this research context, with a focus on how, where, and by whom they were taken up among people in Amuru.

In Amuru sub-county, low saturation of media – including internet access, print media, and even radio – is part of what makes it a different place from the global north where the majority of IE studies have been situated. The forms that texts take are different, and the prevalence of illiteracy contributes to this difference. Some of the bureaucratic texts functioned in ways similar, on the surface, to the forms that govern health care work in Canada, such as the requirement to present a card or a letter at certain times. Less similar was the role of "text-mediated discourses that frame issues, establish terms and concepts" (DeVault & McCoy, 2006, p. 34). These were drawn on by health care providers and administrators and thus played a role in how health care was organized. However, among childbearing women, the discourses framing childbirth and maternity care were mediated very locally, and the role of texts was at times indirect and difficult to trace. For example, MDG 5 or maternal mortality was not part of their discourse and neither were ideas such as "barriers to access," although participants did know that attending a health centre for antenatal and delivery care was encouraged and did speak about barriers, albeit without using such terminology. In the global north, communications technologies have a different use from that which shapes media and bureaucracy in Amuru, where personal computers are unusual, cell phones are common, media consumption is not built into daily lives, and literacy rates are low. Low literacy and a less-saturated media environment influence approaches to care and relationships between patients and providers; the persistence of a relatively paternalistic approach in Amuru restricts to people's ability to be well-informed health care consumers. Adopting IE methods allowed me to explore the role of texts in a low-literacy setting where media and other communications are much less ubiquitous than in the global north.

DISCOURSES

Throughout my analysis, I pay attention to discourses as they are relevant to the social organization of maternity care and birth in Amuru sub-county. Discourses are overarching narratives that have the power to shape social realities. At the same time, people are active in reproducing discourses and can also modify or disrupt them. Drawing from historian of ideas Michel Foucault, Smith (2005) writes that "the functions of 'knowledge, judgment, and will' have become built into a specialized complex of objectified forms of organization and consciousness that organize and coordinate people's everyday lives" (p. 18). Discourses operate at various levels of specificity and influence, with some becoming part of a larger ideology. Smith (2005) explains, "Ideological discourses are generalized and generalizing discourses operating at a metalevel to control other discourses" (p. 224). For example, I argue that through texts, including MDG 5, *maternal mortality* not only refers to the everyday/everynight reality of women dying in childbirth but also is an ideological discourse that influences what can be said and done in relation to maternity care and birth. In an IE approach, discourse is always understood in relation to social actors and activities, as well as to language: it is not of interest until it is activated by being invoked by real people in real places.

## Data Collection

My data collection strategies included interviews and focus groups in two stages, as well as observation and reflexive field notes. During the first stage, I spoke with 45 childbearing women during interviews and focus groups, working with a research assistant (RA) who provided translation. In a second stage, she and I spoke with 22 health workers, with a total of 67 participants in all. These discussions were framed by what I had already learned from the childbearing women and through fieldwork and observation. I had the privilege of working with a committed and knowledgeable RA, Acero (pseudonym), who had experience supporting research and was a trained social worker. She helped to create comfort and rapport with participants, translated questions and responses, and helped to ensure that participants' privacy and informed consent were prioritized. We also spoke at length about cultural norms and language nuances, often on trips to and from the various villages or while waiting for transportation. Before beginning data collection, she trained with me to learn more about IE and qualitative research methods.

In the first stage of interviews and focus groups, I spoke with 45 childbearing women who were age 18 or older, had at least one child under two years old, and were willing to discuss their recent pregnancy, maternity care, and birth. Eighteen is roughly the age at which marrying and having children is accepted within Acholi communities, while those younger might be regarded as taking part in an "early marriage" (Baines & Rosenoff Gauvin, 2014, p. 17). Having a child under two meant that the experiences discussed were relatively recent, to assist in recall, and that the health care women were discussing took place within a similar time frame. Mothers ranged in age from 18 to 41, and had between 1 and 13 children. Residents belonged to similar socio-economic groups; however, for some participants, particularly the wives of leaders, financial concerns were less prominent while other women worried over basics such as daily meals. Most participants were Acholi; two were members of neighbouring ethnic groups who had moved to be with their husbands.[4] Participants were recruited with help from the local leaders, who provided introductions. We then ensured that no participant was too young, as well as ensuring that we did not interview participants married to the same man.

I selected the villages after spending some time in Amuru and with input from local contacts, with a goal of selecting villages that had a range of geographic proximity to care. Proximity to care is an important feature of access, as distance from a health facility shapes various aspects of planning for childbirth. In the parishes of Amuru subcounty, there were 12 villages and four health centres; selecting six villages, two with close proximity to health centres, was a way to capture geographic range. In the interviews, however, I found that people close

---

4 Participants tended not to distinguish between formal marriages and common law or customary partnerships, calling involved male partners "husbands." I have referred to participants' male partners as husbands throughout, in accordance with this practice.

to another health centre actually tended to travel to Lacor HCIII. The prevalence of women with poor geographic access to a health facility in my study is consistent with the circumstances of women in rural northern Uganda. I interviewed 35 women in six villages, and held two focus groups with five participants each at the villages nearest to and farthest from Lacor HCIII.

I was advised that it was essential to introduce myself, my RA, and the project to local leaders; in any case, recognizing local leadership is important to non-colonizing research practices (Smith, 1999). I recruited participants face to face in the villages with the approval of a local leader, either a local council I or a *Rwot Kweri*. Local council (LC) leaders are formal representatives of the government at the local level, while *Rwodi Kweri* (plural form) are male traditional leaders selected by their community on the basis of skill in agriculture. Working with both LC I and *Rwot Kweri* (RK) as village contacts helped ensure a diversity of community size and remoteness. I learned that other researchers who primarily worked through LC I were sometimes limited to the contacts of the LC Is, to the exclusion of the RKs' contacts, who were often more remotely located. Being able to speak with women in remote locations, partly as a result of my association with the RKs, helped me gain a fuller picture of the contexts of maternity care and childbirth in the sub-county. I sat down with each village leader to discuss the goal of our visit to their village, how long we would be there, and with whom I would be talking. At the end of our time in each village, I asked leaders to share with us anything they thought we should know about birth and maternity care in their area, conversations that often ended up being extensive in scope. LC leaders and RKs talked to us about the wide range of local issues that affected maternal health, which, depending on location, included transportation, HIV, land appropriation, and so on. They shared stories of maternal deaths, including one that had particularly unsettled people and that we heard several times, about a woman who died during a footling breach birth and was buried with the baby partially born. Alongside the loss of lives, the inability to properly bury the dead was unsettling to those who shared this story.

I asked participants to select the interview location, and we spoke in their hut, a community space such as a church, or, most often, a shaded outdoor area. Before each interview, we spent some time explaining the research and its goals and reviewing and signing consent forms, often with a thumb print, at the preference of participants' who struggled to write their name. We demonstrated the voice recorders and explained their purpose. Participants brought their smaller children to sit with them for the interviews, and Acero also brought her young son along for fieldwork, meaning that there were often not one but two babies in each interview. His presence helped establish that the visiting researchers were also mothers. We paused for small interruptions so participants could help their children. I introduced myself as a mother and researcher, and explained where I was from and that I was not a nurse or health worker (in case any part of our interaction was misunderstood as a health visit). My own preschool-age son did not accompany us when leaving the village, but when he was curious about a focus group held with health workers near our home, he sat with us for a while.

During interviews, I asked open-ended questions, including "What does *maternal health* mean to you?" and "What do you do to prepare for childbirth?" Such questions provided an opportunity for the participants to produce narratives that explained their experience of birth and care, including the activities and work in relation to care, and for them to give detailed examples of the strengths and challenges in local support for childbirth. Acero provided translation and helped suggest follow-up questions. My intention was for the interviews to focus primarily on the birth of the youngest child, under two years of age at the time of the interviews. While this remained the primary focus, when women were pregnant at the time of the interviews, or had had several children in close succession, a broader focus on their experiences was introduced. This happened when participants were keen to share information about their current or recent pregnancies or to compare one recent experience with another. This flexible approach to interview content is consistent with IE approaches to interviewing, in which interviews are "an open-ended inquiry" (DeVault & McCoy, 2006, p. 23).

Focus groups are a method that shifts the balance of power towards participants (Wilkinson 1998, p. 282) in part because such groups are often situated in a social context in which participants are comfortable. It was clear that focus group participants were relaxed and enjoyed the opportunity to discuss these matters together. While the interview setting was appropriate for women's private experiences, fears, and concerns, the focus groups sometimes tended towards a more general discussion of the issues, with support for those women who shared personal stories. Overall, there was a strong feeling of solidarity within the focus groups: a lot of laughter at a backwards walking chicken contrasting with the quiet supportive listening as women recounted their more difficult experiences of conflict and loss. My guiding questions for these focus groups were developed based on responses to the initial interviews.

As well as interviewing mothers, I conducted focus groups and interviews with 22 health workers involved in maternity care, such as VHT members, TBAs,[5] and health care centre medical staff (nurses and midwives). I included this research stage based on the IE practice of looking "up and out" from one's initial site of inquiry into institutional practices that shape that initial site. This second stage acts as an opportunity for a researcher to "begin examining those institutional practices that he or she has discovered to be shaping the experience but that are not wholly known to the original informants" (DeVault & McCoy, 2006, p. 21). While the formal elements of recording talk with childbearing women and then with health workers were sequential, since I was living at the health centre, I was learning from health workers all the time. Our informal conversations and the trips we took together contributed to my knowledge of how care was organized. Some of the health worker participants lived in staff housing too; our children played together and we spoke often. Others, in particular VHT members, were people I had met only briefly or not at all before the interview.

I used a broad and encompassing definition of care providers, rather than focusing solely on either formal health care providers or informal care providers. This was because both employees of the formal health system and people working at the village level, such as TBAs and members of the VHT, were likely to play a significant role, because their roles might overlap, and because, at the outset of research, it was unknown whether childbearing women in Amuru made a clear distinction between formal and informal sources of maternity care and labour support. As it transpired, birthing women did tend to refer to a large and varied group of health workers as *daktari*, a Swahili[6] word meaning "doctor." The health workers, whether formal or lay, all also worked to farm land, often alongside another side occupation; most were also parents, and, particularly in the case of TBAs, grandparents.

The goal of the focus groups and interviews with health workers was to explore the link between mothers' insights into how support for childbirth is coordinated and the work processes of those involved in providing health support for birthing women. I asked general questions so that health workers could describe the care they provided and any challenges they met in providing it, but the primary focus of the interviews was determined by the contents of the initial interviews with birthing women. For

---

5 Recently, practising TBAs have been required to be VHT members. Women make up a minority of the VHT; among them, many are TBAs.

6 While the mother tongue of the Acholi is Acholi (Luo), widely spoken throughout northern Uganda, English is the official language of Uganda with Swahili also voted as an official language (though not ratified). Swahili is widely understood in east Africa, and people sometimes use Swahili loan-words when speaking other languages.

example, some women had reported giving birth at the health centre but unattended by health centre staff, so I asked health workers about whether this happened and what might lead to such circumstances.

I spoke with one focus group of five general members of the VHT and two focus groups of five TBAs (who were also VHT members). These focus groups were held in Acholi, with members introducing some commentary in English. We talked at the health centre after meetings that had occasioned a gathering of VHT or TBAs from the sub-county; we sat outside on benches or in a roofed area, depending on the weather. Among formal care providers, I interviewed two nurses; the clinical officer in-charge, the public health educator, the district health officer (DHO), and two midwives. Interviews with formal care providers were held in English, at their preference. All participants in both stages are referred to by pseudonyms throughout; most Acholi people are known by two given names: an Acholi name and another name that is often biblical or European. The pseudonyms selected are not Acholi but are names that would plausibly be a given name.

As part of my fieldwork while I was in Amuru, I kept a journal that was a combination of field notes and reflexive writing. I tracked observations and talk related to maternity care and birth, or other areas of social life as they appeared relevant. I wrote about my own role and relationships as researcher. For example, I was curious about a rumour that circulated that I was breastfeeding my son, then four or five. I finally realized it pertained to the prevalence of breastfeeding as a means of child spacing and the fact that he was so old for a single child. As Smith (2014) writes, "There is constant leakage from the multivoiced society in which we do our work into our sociological work" (p. 234). Reflexivity is a means of understanding how our analyses are shaped by circulating discourses. A guiding principal during fieldwork was that "data are everywhere"; the journal was a place where I had free rein to consider observations without having to make a decision about whether they were ultimately significant parts of my data or analysis. I worked out initial analyses, which I then discussed with my RA or others. These field notes help to form an audit trail as I could see when certain analyses began to emerge. For example, in two entries at the end of May, I was critical of responsibilization practices around public health messaging generally and on malaria in particular. I wrote, "Some of the health messaging that people wear on their backs [i.e., on T-shirts], like 'eradicate neglected disease' – well, who are they talking to? The poor people in these villages are not the ones who can eradicate them." This insight that certain practices shift responsibility towards individuals and away from social structures informed my analysis of the social organization of maternity care and childbirth.

In these field notes, I wrote about being called over to an outdoor area at the health centre to meet newborn twins; their mother's joy and desire to share it was evident. Another day, I saw a woman leaving the health centre with a baby on her back and an even smaller baby in her arms. Her sister had died in childbirth and since she was already nursing her own baby, she was adopting the newborn. These women were not formally part of the study, yet my encounters with their everyday joys and hardships shaped my understanding of care and birth in the area. This immersion in the field contrasts with typical IE practices in which researchers live at home while visiting a site for interviews, observations, or other research practices. Overlapping IE practices with other critical ethnographic practices broadened the lens of study, allowing for a clear and complex picture of the organization of maternity care and birth.

Because I was required to seek ethics approval at three levels in Uganda, as well as at my home university, part of my research experience included a waiting period. Mannay and Morgan (2014) write about how, despite the temptation for researchers to "rush into the field armed with audio recorder and camera" (p. 4), there is an often overlooked value in "the waiting field," which they describe as "'spaces previous to,' 'spaces of interruption/disruption' and 'spaces of reflection'" (p. 7). During this time, I familiarized myself with the area, learned how to manage day-to-day life in this new setting, and developed relationships with health centre staff and neighbours. I had long talks with ambulance drivers who gave me a ride to Gulu town when transporting patients, telling me their stories as we bumped along the dirt road at high speed. Living in staff housing, I was able to witness a five-and-a-half day workweek transform into a seven day workweek because of an outreach trip, chat with the midwives while they sat outside their rooms of an evening cutting up plastic sheeting for deliveries, and, when I heard the distinctive roar of the ambulance late at night, get the story the next morning.

My primary observation site was at the health centre, which is where most care to pregnant women of Amuru took place and where the health workers spent most of their working, and indeed private, lives. However, my extended period of fieldwork also allowed for serendipitous opportunities, such as observing outreach to all areas of the sub-county, sitting in on an NGO program delivering nutrition education, and seeing the training dolls given to TBAs (despite the lack of international support for TBA training). When I did not have interviews scheduled, I took every opportunity to observe outreach, program delivery, or health talks in an effort to understand the full scope of practices and interactions around care. I accompanied a team of health workers to an isolated village on the Nile, where they provided vitamins and deworming tablets and conducted antenatal check-ups. I observed the midwives setting up their antenatal station and chatting with groups of patients. I wrote about this as follows:

> The first village we went to was a longish drive (1 hour and half, going fast by ambulance) and then a quite long walk in (maybe 45 minutes) on a steep single track trail. Quite pretty. [Description of greetings, vaccinations, etc.] We also went on a short boat ride in the dugout canoes – they were making them, and spear-shaped paddles, right there. We paddled out of a little sheltered area in the reeds, and onto a calm section of the Nile. The village itself seemed very poor: the houses were in bad repair, and one home was just a central ridge pole with a tarp – others were this same tent shape but with thatch. A few of the children had distended bellies with swollen, protruding belly buttons. The villagers sold dried fish to some of the health workers, and were busy patching their fishing nets. Lots of small plastic bags for vodka were littering the path. But also, there was an area where we collected wild tamarind just off the path ... A district engineer had been a week prior (according to their guest book) and was looking at building road access to the Nile.

The opportunity to observe outreach helped me get familiar not just with health care strategies, but also with the differing social circumstances of people in the sub-county.

Although the midwives invited me to make myself at home in the labour suite, I felt that this would be intrusive and that meaningful consent would be difficult to negotiate, so I did not observe any births. I came across training manuals, posters, and brochures that were part of the environment at the health centre or at offices I visited, the analysis of which became part of the research. (This was in addition to my formal review of the policy and academic literature.) These aspects of fieldwork extended the lens of the other more formal data collection methods.

In addition to formal academic dissemination of the research, such as publications and conference presentations, I shared the initial findings of the research with community members, including health centre administrators and local leaders, in a verbal report and discussion. I also sent my draft study to senior administrators at the hospital and health centre, as well as the DHO, and invited their input.

*Positioning Myself as Researcher*

I first became interested in the needs of mothers and children in post-conflict settings when working in Thailand at a home for children in

2004. Most of the hundred children who lived there had fled conflict and displacement in neighbouring Burma. I struggled to accept the injustices these children had faced and, in particular, could not reconcile my anger over one child, a popular boy of eight, who had AIDS. Despite my growing understanding of the economic and social impacts of the conflict, my anger was directed towards his mother, who sold sex near the border and whose rare visits her son proudly anticipated. I knew that I needed to push past this visceral emotion to a clearer analysis of the conditions that had led to his illness and abandonment, and eventually to his death. Through the stories shared by young residents and by the human rights activists who were our neighbours, I learned about the impacts of the conflict on families of surviving violence, poverty, displacement, and statelessness. When I worked on a gender-based violence research project in South Africa, at the Center for the Study of Violence and Reconciliation, I was struck by how similar certain challenges were to those of displaced Burmese people, despite the different historical and cultural settings. My commitment to research on respectful and safe reproductive and sexual health care continues to cross national contexts.

*Theorizing Methods*

To adequately consider relational ethics for this project, I needed to draw on methodological approaches that explicitly resist the colonizing potential of research in addition to IE research methods. Smith (2005) "rejects the dominance of theory" in sociological inquiry (p. 49); this rejection means that IE "findings are not already prejudged by a conceptual framework that regulates how data will be interpreted" (Smith, 2005, p. 50). The rejection of reliance on theory can be understood as a form of methodological bracketing (Hussey, 2012). Hussey explains:

> The researcher makes the ontological shift to reject speculative explanations. This involves a move away from general and generalizing theoretical explanations to a particular, embodied, situated, "sensuous world of people's actual practices and activities" ([Smith,] 1990: 633). This technique of bracketing ideological procedures implores the researcher to focus analysis on explicating temporal-spatial-situational actualities ([Smith,] 1990: 637–638). (p. 9)

With these critiques of reliance on theory in mind, I have used social justice as an important touchstone, drawn from non-colonizing methodologies, and implemented intersectionality theory and methodology to best attend to the contexts of participants' lives.

The term *transnational* is useful for understanding how health policy and practices are organized in global south settings. In labelling this field of health interventions, there has been a movement from *tropical medicine* or *international health*, terms associated with practices during the colonial era, to *global health* (Adams, 2010; Biehl & Petryna, 2013). *Global health* is now the dominant term used to refer to the transnational implementation of health care practices and policies, an implementation that still often flows north-south; less frequently, it refers to a field of academic study. By way of definition, Rieder (2016) suggests understanding global health "as a set of complex processes that occur in specific places at the intersections of multiple transnational networks and are best studied within the fraught interactions of human and non-human actors, technologies, and institutions" (p. 56). The term *global health* has an optimistic ring; Dilger and Mattes (2018) advocate for a shift from global health to "medical globalization" to acknowledge the power relations at play. In employing the term *transnational* in this book, I am similarly interested in complex power relations that move across national boundaries and also between administrative levels, from high-level international organizing such as at the WHO to local decision making in settings like Amuru.

The term *local* may also require elaboration. Janes and Corbett (2009) suggest that for ethnographers, who are interested "people-in-contexts," Ginsburg and Rapp's (1995, as cited in Janes & Corbett, 2009) definition is useful: "The local is not defined by geographical boundaries but is understood as any small-scale arena in which social meanings are informed and adjusted" (p. 169). Similarly, I use *local* to refer to the immediate geographic and social circle of the participants in Amuru.

Adequate support during pregnancy is a social justice concern. Theories of social justice challenge us to identify the root source of inequities within complex social and power structures (Hankivsky et al., 2012, p. 38). A capabilities approach to social justice makes the case that people's ability to engage in practical freedoms is central to well-being, alongside the material goods that are the focus of distributive justice (Sen, 1999). Nussbaum (2000, 2003) created a list of central capabilities, including life, bodily health, bodily integrity, and the political and material control of one's environment, among others (Nussbaum, 2000). As explored by Iris Marion Young (2008), there is a tension between these social justice approaches and the individual focus of much human rights discourse. Young (2008) suggests a turn towards relationships and social groups as central to justice.

Central to social justice contexts in Uganda is colonialism; as with other areas of social interaction, research and scholarship has a colonial legacy, and its practices have been influenced by postcolonial and decolonizing theorizing. Various scholars have examined the connections between the practices of academic research and ongoing colonialism (Browne et al., 2005; Mohanty, 1988, 2013; Smith, 1999), while others have tried to identify and develop research practices that can be decolonizing. For example, Linda T. Smith (1999) makes the case that qualitative research is a valuable tool for Indigenous communities, for its power to "situate, place, and contextualize," to "create spaces for decolonizing," and to "understand little and big changes that affect our lives" (p. 136). In a consideration of the value of postcolonial studies to health care research, Browne et al. (2005) write that

> a postcolonial interpretation locates health and social conditions in the domain of the historical and structural disadvantages that shape them. From the selection and framing of research questions, to decisions on the dissemination and presentation of findings, vigilance is required, in order to decrease the potential for research processes to undermine our broader transformative goals. (p. 31)

Such insights advance a potentially transformative agenda in addressing power dynamics between academic researchers and communities struggling with poverty and poor resources.

As well as looking to social justice and non-colonizing research practices to help ensure ethical research, I draw on intersectionality, an approach developed by Kimberlé Crenshaw (1991) that examines how multiple social and structural factors overlap and constitute systematic power relationships based on oppression and privilege. Intersectionality "requires a consideration of the complex relationship between mutually constituting factors of social location and structural disadvantage so as to more accurately map and conceptualize determinants of equity and inequity in and beyond health" (Hankivsky et al., 2012, p. 18). As Weber (2006) writes, within intersectionality, "inequalities are conceived as social constructions situated in social contexts and structures beyond the individual – in societies, institutions, communities, and families – and are characterized as power, not simply resource, difference between dominant and subordinate groups" (p. 24). An intersectional approach is consistent with a social justice approach to research and helps to understand relations of gender and power.

While social justice, decolonizing research methodology, and intersectionality helped to guide this research from the outset, structural violence and responsibilization are theoretical concepts whose significance to the project emerged later, as I was working with initial data and on analysis. These are ideas that I have returned to repeatedly in working through my understanding of multiple facets of the findings. I offer a brief description here.

*Structural violence* is a term coined by the Norwegian sociologist Johan Galtung (1969). I first came across it in the work of medical anthropologist Paul Farmer of Partners in Health, whose advocacy for health care that meets the needs of the poor has challenged mainstream approaches to global health. Among scholars of the conflict in northern Uganda, the concept is frequently used to indicate the myriad ways the violence of the war extended beyond instrumental violence (e.g., Annan & Brier, 2010; Branch, 2013; Finnström, 2008; Westerhaus et al., 2007). Farmer (2010) describes structural violence as follows:

> "Structural violence" is one way of describing social arrangements marked by racism and other social inequalities. In the influential view of sociologist Johan Galtung, structural violence is "the avoidable impairment of fundamental human needs, embedded in longstanding ubiquitous social structures, normalized by stable institutions and regular experience." Because they seem so ordinary in our ways of understanding the world, such violent structures are almost invisible. Disparate access to resources, political power, and health care as well as unequal legal standing are just a few examples. Such arrangements do violence to society's losers; the arrangements are structural because they are embedded in the economic organization of our social world. (p. 578)

For Galtung (1969), an "extended concept of violence is indispensable" to having a meaningful understanding of peace (p. 158) so that social injustices are prioritized alongside ending personal violence. In studies of health and health care, the concept of structural violence can, alongside models such as the social determinants of health, act as a corrective to an overreliance on biomedical models of health, in which the primary location for understanding poor health is the body. The social structures that produce inequities – colonization, patriarchy and gender discrimination, economic disparities – have a layering effect, the result of which can coalesce in structural violence.

Responsibilization is another concept that was key in helping me to understand the social relations around care. In the journal *Health, Risk and Society,* I wrote about how the neoliberal discourse of taking charge of one's own health, familiar from Western media and public health efforts, was also present in northern Uganda (Rudrum, 2017). Such calls to healthy living depend on discourses of choice and responsibility, as "citizens individually are assumed to be able to assist in the task of governance through acting 'responsibly,' taking appropriate preventive action and exercising 'informed choice' in the burgeoning biomedical market-place" (Petersen et al., 2010, p. 395). Nicholas Rose (2007) clearly situates the problem as specific to particular political contexts prevalent in the global north when he writes, "This complex of marketization, autonomization, and responsibilization gives a particular character to the contemporary politics of life in advanced liberal democracies" (p. 2). The social and political context for health care in northern Uganda departs greatly from the contexts that the responsibilization critique was developed in response to; certainly the marketplace for health-related consumption is hardly burgeoning. However, calls to responsibilization were evident in various sites: the training (and rationale) for the VHTs, the incentivizing of delivery care via gifts, and the requirement for women to bring a husband to test for HIV during ANC, for example. The presence of neoliberal responsibilization practices in this remote health care setting speaks to the long reach of global health practices and the way in which they carry ideologies with them; these practices and ideologies are shaped disproportionately by the global north, where the money, decision making, and more generally, power are concentrated. A central feature of responsibilization as a critique of approaches to health and health care is that its discourse of individual responsibility simultaneously absolves structures and institutions from responsibility for health (Petersen et al., 2010; Rossiter, 2012). It became clear through the research that many of the problems surrounding maternity care would be best solved, in Uganda as elsewhere in countries with weak health systems, by the (deceptively) straightforward investment in health care – in clinics, staff, and supplies. I make the case that, in various ways, responsibilization messages and strategies surrounding health detracted from a focus on the health system.

## Outline

This book comprises six chapters including this introductory chapter. Chapter 2 scopes the history and aftermath of the protracted conflict between the LRA and government forces, and makes the case that the post-conflict context is one of ongoing social distress. Causes of this distress include insecure land tenure amid corporate and government expansion in the region and the fear of disease outbreak. As well as poor infrastructure and inadequate investment, social distress affects maternity care and approaches to pregnancy and birth. The health consequences of conflict, displacement, and post-conflict are intertwined with the social and political consequences. Social justice and health care access are interwoven: "Receiving health care, not receiving health care, and how health care is offered all affect physical health and at the same time carry messages about citizenship" (Sinding, 2010, p. 1657). Finnström (2008) articulates how such messages may work in his book about the meaning of the conflict in everyday life in northern Uganda, *Living with Bad Surroundings: War, History, and Everyday Moments in Northern Uganda.* Chris Dolan (2009) argues that the war, including the internal displacement camps, constituted *social torture.* These recurring violations occurring under the guise of protection are also pursued in Branch's (2011) book *Displacing Human Rights: War and Intervention in Northern Uganda,* which focuses on the role of humanitarian intervention. My fieldwork took place in the year of the controversial KONY 2012 social media campaign that called for 2012 to be the year in which international forces collaborated to capture LRA leader Joseph Kony. I discuss the controversies surrounding this campaign, previewing NGO-community tensions in the region, a theme of chapter 4.

Chapter 3 offers a background on how approaches to care and birth in Amuru, northern Uganda, were structured by everyday challenges associated with poverty and lack of infrastructure, the most prominent of which were having access to transportation, avoiding arduous physical work while pregnant, and ensuring adequate nutrition. Chapter 3 provides a narrative of the everyday in which care was sought, as well as offering a critical overview of the informal and formal health services available to pregnant women.

Chapter 4 describes how a gift to new mothers from an international and national NGO was leveraged as an incentive to care. The mama kit reproduced discourses about scarcity, responsibility, and deservingness while shaping approaches to organizing care. A participant described the gift as "the help they give when they've seen how different you are" and suggested that it was a poor substitute for the health care services and transportation infrastructure required to support safe delivery. Chapter 4 draws on critical approaches to international development to demonstrate that, rather than representing a one-way flow of goods and altruism, charitable gifts in fact bind the global north and global south in complex ways.

Chapter 5's focus is HIV prevention during maternity care. I examine the effects of a compulsory approach to couples' HIV testing, the testing of pregnant women and their husbands during ANC. I identify the strategies via which the test was presented as mandatory, one of which was to assert that delivery care was contingent on presenting a test result. I trace the impacts of testing protocols. In the context of some husbands' reluctance to test, the approach to testing contributed to the potential for intimate partner violence, as well as impacting future care, particularly delivery care. I make the case that a "vertical" approach by international health bodies, in which health issues, including HIV and maternity care, are addressed as silos rather than through comprehensive health services or "horizontal" approaches, puts the goal of HIV reduction in competition with the goal of reducing maternal mortality. These findings are particularly relevant because of policy contexts in which compulsory approaches are being formalized, such as through Uganda's *HIV and AIDS Prevention and Control Act, 2014* (Republic of Uganda, 2014). This type of legislation, becoming more common throughout the region, criminalizes HIV transmission and compels health workers to disclose patients' HIV status, alongside making HIV testing mandatory for pregnant women and their intimate partners or spouses. Such coercive approaches are a threat to adequate health care and to human rights more broadly.

The book's concluding chapter reflects on the various failures of intervention identified in earlier chapters, returning from the case of northern Uganda to the larger issue of how global health discourses and practices typically frame the crisis in maternal health and its solutions. The twin tendencies to govern via large-scale standardized public health interventions shaped by global north technocracies while blaming local culture, tradition, and social relations for poor health outcomes are pervasive within research and practice on the maternal health crisis in global south countries with high ratios of maternal mortality. Standardizing and colonizing tendencies manifest in a focus on barriers to access to care and on cultural preference, also labelled tradition. When the maternal health challenge is attributed to access barriers plus cultural norms, the institutional practices that produce the politics and practices of maternity care are neglected. These institutional practices are complex, as they are simultaneously transnational and highly localized in scope, but need to be understood to better understand the present challenge in maternal health.

In the chapters that follow, I examine the unique interplay between post-conflict recovery, NGO engagement, and global health governance in northern Uganda as they shape maternity care. Alongside the challenges inherent in accessing care in a resource-poor area within a weak health system, approaches to coordinating care are influenced by global health initiatives and their long but clumsy reach. Using northern Uganda as a case, I extrapolate to more widely applicable insights about how global health currently operates, making the argument that poor outcomes of global health interventions are often as labelled "unintended consequences" but are better understood as resulting from specific problems in how maternal health challenges are framed and approached.

# Chapter Two

# Ongoing Social Distress: Care Seeking in a Remote Post-conflict Context

## Introduction

Long years of war between the government's Uganda People's Defence Force (UPDF) and the LRA, a group of rebels led by Joseph Kony, have impacted every aspect of life for surviving Acholi people, including health, health care, and childbirth. This chapter provides an overview of the conflict and outlines its ongoing social and economic impacts as they shape life and as they affect birthing women and access to care in Amuru sub-county. Aspects of the conflict, such as abduction and forced displacement, have ongoing significance for all parts of life, including health broadly and reproductive health specifically, in the post-conflict period. I explore the social distress caused by the outbreak and potential outbreak of disease and by land disputes, arguing that these are sites of an ongoing struggle for inclusion and justice. The post-conflict period has been a time of flux; people have been returning home, and multiple overlapping interventions from government and NGOs have shaped the local infrastructure as it relates to health care. This detailed contextual account sets the stage for the findings that are particular to maternity care in Amuru.

## Overview of the Conflict in Northern Uganda

Described as a "dirty war" for its targeting of civilians and use of terror as means of warfare (Finnström, 2008), the conflict between the LRA in northern Uganda and government forces spanned over two decades and still continues outside Uganda's borders. The war was characterized by the abduction of children, mass forced displacement, and the indiscriminate killing of civilians (Branch, 2011; Dolan, 2009; Finnström, 2008). These violations have left the economic and social dimensions of Acholi life deeply damaged, with adverse consequences for women's health.

The population of Acholiland is primarily rural; outside of towns, subsistence agriculture is the primary means of making a living among the Acholi, a predominantly Christian group. Since the internal displaced people (IDP) camps were disbanded, most residents had by 2012, my fieldwork period, returned to their rural homes and were once again farming and keeping livestock, though to a more limited extent than before the conflict. Amuru is a relatively new district, created in 2005 and formerly part of Gulu district. This area is north of Murchison Falls National Park and south of the border with South Sudan, extending to West Nile and, in the east, to Gulu district, where Gulu town is a bustling regional centre. I undertook this research in a sub-county within the district, also called Amuru, while based in staff housing at Lacor HCIII, Amuru, located at a disbanded IDP camp where some crumbling camp infrastructure, such as signage and tap-stands, remained.

It can be difficult to identify a clear starting point of the conflict (Dolan, 2009, p. 39), and to identify its roots, one must look to the colonial period. A British protectorate since 1894, Uganda gained independence in 1962. British administrators had relied on a "divide-and-rule strategy" (Dolan, 2009, p. 41), which included the consolidation of oppositional ethnic identities. During this period, the Bagandan people residing in the south were accorded economic and political power as farmers and civil servants, while the Acholi were recruited into the military and into manual labour. During the colonial period, "no one group or sub-region enjoyed both military and economic power simultaneously, and discourses of ethnic difference were established which live on to this day" (Dolan 2009, p. 42). While the distribution of power under the British and since has contributed to conflict, a view of the LRA/UPDF conflict as stemming primarily from a priori ethnic tensions is both inaccurate and prejudiced.

Upon independence, the role of Acholi people on the national scene shifted in relation to the various postcolonial national governments. Under the brutal regime of Idi Amin (1971–9), Acholi people were the targets of mass killings, ostensibly as reprisal for their association with the prior prime minister, Milton Obote. When Obote came to power again, this time as president (Obote II, 1980–5), Acholi people were once again better represented in the armed forces. Ending the brief presidency (July 1985 to January 1986) of Tito Okello, an Acholi general, Yoweri Museveni took power in January 1986, by defeating the Acholi-dominated Uganda National Liberation Army (NLA) with his National Resistance Army (NRA) in a violent insurgency (Finnström, 2008). Museveni remains president more than 30 years later (as of 2021).

The year 1986 also marked the start of the rebel movement. In March 1986, Museveni's NRA had "reached and taken Gulu," the major town of the north (Dolan, 2009, p. 43). Resistance to the NRA's violent occupation, and its practice of stealing cattle, came from the Ugandan People's Democratic Army (UPDA), made up of soldiers of the former regime. Opposition also came from Alice Auma, known as Alice Lakwena, meaning "messenger," and her Holy Spirit Movement (HSM). A spirit medium and healer, Lakwena became a military leader to recruits who shared her goal of overthrowing Museveni's National Resistance Movement government and forming an inclusive and non-violent government. The HSM under Lakwena was a short-lived military force; the group was overpowered at Jinja by the NRA on an attempted incursion to the capital, Kampala, in October 1987. A peace accord was signed with the UPDA in 1988, but rebel movements opposing the government persisted. The HSM continued under Alice Lakwena's father, Severino Lukwoya, while she herself fled to Kenya. It was at this time that Joseph Kony became leader of the northern rebels, calling his group the LRA and, like Lakwena, basing his claim to leadership on spiritual authority. Kony led the LRA throughout the rest of the long conflict in northern Uganda and continues to lead a diminished LRA operating in neighbouring countries. After some initial support, quite quickly Kony was "confronted with a deficit of volunteers, a population unwilling to support continued violence, and a number of different opponents" (Branch, 2011, p. 68). Initial NRA responses were harsh: homes and granaries were destroyed by fire, and many people were killed (Dolan, 2009).

While the conflict pitted Kony's army against Museveni's, civilians were the main victims, with assailants and perpetrators originating on both sides. Various features of the war, including the abduction of children into the LRA, the arming of civilians by the UPDF, and the constant threat of being branded as either a rebel or a supporter of the government, blurred the distinction between civilians and combatants (Finnström, 2008, p. 89). Attacks on civilians occurred in LRA reprisals for lack of support and, in turn, contributed to a lack of support. The LRA's large-scale abduction, maiming, and attacking of civilians perhaps contributed to a view that they operated without a coherent political or military agenda; however, the group did make political demands (Finnström, 2008).

By the mid-1990s, a practice of internal displacement began, partly in response to increased targeting of Acholi civilians by the LRA, in apparent resentment for their lack of support and their perceived collaboration with government forces (Dolan, 2009, p. 45). The majority of the population of Acholiland, some 1.8 million people, was eventually displaced into these camps (McElroy et al., 2012). A series of massacres and mass abductions in 1995 and 1996 heightened the terror. Many people, especially children, began a practice of "night commuting," walking to safer areas to sleep communally and returning to their homes, schools, or gardens by day (Dolan, 2009, p. 46). Lacor Hospital, near Gulu, which operated the health centre where I lived and whose work is discussed throughout this book, was a major host to night commuters, accommodating thousands of people, even tens of thousands at the peak of the insurgency in 2002 (Lacor Hospital, n.d.-a, p. 2). A survival strategy, night commuting placed pressure on families and contributed to the breakdown of protective social structures (Falk et al., 2004). In late 1996, the government created the first IDP camps, which it identified as "protected villages." Some residents willingly left their homes, where they feared attacks or abductions, but removal to the camps became increasingly forcible. In 2002, the UPDF's Operation Iron Fist escalated fighting against the LRA and expanded forced displacement. The "protection" the government promised did not materialize; the presence of the UPDF was minimal in the camps, and these soldiers seldom fought back against LRA attacks. Abductions and attacks continued in the camps. In 1994, peace talks were held but failed. Each side blamed the other, with Museveni's demand that LRA forces surrender within a week remembered as particularly damaging (Branch, 2011, p. 74, Dolan, 2009, p. 46; Finnström, 2008, p. 89).

While the conflict has often been understood as local and ethnic, major powers were also involved. The LRA was bolstered from the early 1990s by support from Sudan, and in return assisted in Khartoum's fight against south Sudanese rebels (Finnström, 2008, p. 84). Other global features of the war included extensive international humanitarian aid to the IDP camps, the United States' listing of the LRA as a terrorist group in 2001, and the International Criminal Court's identification of Kony and other LRA commanders as wanted war criminals in 2005. (In 2015, the International Criminal Court charged LRA commander Dominic Ongwen with crimes against humanity despite the fact that he was "recruited" via abduction as a child; Baines (2009) has explored Ongwen's case as that of a "complex political perpetrator" (p. 180), noting that it may be exceptional in charging someone with "the war crimes of which he was also a victim" (pp. 163–164).) Branch (2011) makes a detailed case that international humanitarian aid facilitated the government's strategy of forcible displacement and was otherwise harmful to the Acholi people, while Finnström (2008) argues that it was "indeed a global war" despite being "fought on local grounds" (p. 9). International military assistance to both sides, and humanitarian assistance to civilians, complicated the conflict but did little to resolve it.

A cessation of hostilities agreement between the LRA and the government was signed and renewed at the Juba Peace Talks in 2006 ("Agreement on Cessation of Hostilities," 2006; (Dolan, 2009). However, Kony refused to sign the final agreement in 2008, leaving lingering doubt as to whether peace in Acholiland would last. Dating the end to armed conflict to the time of the Juba Peace Talks is only possible retrospectively. At the time of this writing, Kony is still at large, leading a smaller army in hostilities in countries neighbouring Uganda.

## Ongoing Social and Economic Impacts of the War

The conflict brought great social and economic devastation to Acholi people. Its impacts were highly gendered and changed family dynamics, work responsibilities, and approaches to health care for women. In examining these social and economic repercussions, I focus on two events experienced by many Acholi people: abduction and internment. The war years led to the destruction of people's livelihoods, alongside their witnessing the atrocities of war, leading Dolan (2009) to refer to the period of the conflict as an overall reversal of fortunes for the Acholi people. Abduction and displacement were two aspects of the conflict that make a return to normalcy in the aftermath of violence difficult. They have lasting harms that impact maternity care and birth, in terms of both individual needs and social supports.

### Abduction, Health, and Community Membership

Over 60,000 children and youth were abducted during the war (Baines & Stewart, 2011; Westerhaus, 2007). Fewer girls than boys were abducted (Annan et al., 2011); among the abducted children, between 15 and 30 per cent were girls (Austin et al., 2008; Corbin, 2008; Pham et al., 2012). The experience of girl abductees, which I focus on here, provides a narrow entry point into a complex social reality and demonstrates the direct connection between abduction and women's lives and reproductive health. However, it is important to recognize that boys and men experienced wide-ranging violence that impaired their physical, mental, and social well-being, and that this harm in turn contributed to the social and material context in which women seek care.

Girls and women who were abducted and forced to travel, live, and fight with the LRA faced specific and ongoing impacts to their health, including their sexual and reproductive health. While the development of consensual relationships among abductees was not permitted, girls were "given" to, or forced to "marry," commanders. Erin Baines (2014), a political scientist who has worked with former abductee members of the Women's Advocacy Network, argues that "against the backdrop of deprivation and coercion in which it took place" forced marriage and motherhood also "became an important strategy of survival as well as a means to achieve a position of authority" (p. 414). In addition to the trauma of abduction and forced marriage, forced sex left girls and women susceptible to pregnancy (Omona & Aduo, 2013) and to infections, including gonorrhea, syphilis, and HIV. The conditions of abduction and armed conflict made pregnancies dangerous and motherhood precarious. Some complications and infections led to permanent gynecological problems (Mazurana et al., 2002, p. 114). Women's experiences of forced marriage and other sexual violence have an ongoing impact on their well-being and their reproductive health.

Evelyn Amony, who was forced to marry LRA leader Joseph Kony and spent four years in LRA custody, bearing four children, recounts the circumstances of her marriage and her life as an LRA abductee. She writes (Amony & Shaya, 2012):

> We were constantly on the move, running and hiding from the UPDF, crossing rivers and walking miles, often with injuries. After giving birth, it became more difficult for me to keep up with my unit … I had to carry one child on my back and other children in my arms, all while carrying luggage on my head. I watched several of my friends die as a result of bombs being dropped during combat by the UPDF soldiers. (para. 3)

For abducted women, giving birth was one in a sequence of traumatic events and brought new challenges, as well as joy and meaning.

In addition to the health consequences of abduction, the returnees and their children have faced social consequences after living among the rebels. Amony (2015; Amony & Shaya, 2012) describes how women's ability to adjust after returning is hindered by stigma directed towards them and their children. She elaborates that this stigmatization can include the rejection of returnees, who are often blamed for what they did while in LRA custody and who may not be seen as innocent victims. Community members may fear that formerly abducted people will be possessed by *cen,* "vengeance ghosts" (P'Bitek, 1971, p. 55) or "polluting spirits" (Allen, 2007; Porter, 2012) that can disrupt the social world, and whose presence therefore requires a social solution (Allen, 2007). Stigma and ostracism mean that women have diminished access to the family support, both social and economic, that they rely on to have a healthy pregnancy, seek care, and raise children.

As a result of stigmatization, those returning from abduction after conflicts sometimes form new household arrangements after kin have rejected them (Austin et al., 2008). In the case of Uganda, international NGOs have contributed to stigma by misreporting on the sexual experiences of girl abductees. Initial reports suggested that girls were forced into "promiscuous" sex with multiple commanders, whereas it was more often the case that they were forced into serial-monogamous or polygynous marriages (Spittal et al., 2008). This misunderstanding, and the harms it led to for women attempting to reintegrate, points to the importance of understanding the specific consequences of the post-conflict context. Amony identifies the misperception that if you are abducted, men "sleep with you just anyhow" as a motivation to write her memoir about life after abduction (Amony, 2015, p. xii).

### The Internally Displaced Persons (IDP) Camps

While the camps were initially euphemistically referred to as protected villages, the forcible displacement of the majority of Acholi civilians was a military strategy intended to cut off the supply of food and soldiers to the rebels, who raided, abducted, and were sometimes voluntarily supported by civilians. The camps were a location of structural violence, a concept describing social arrangements based in inequity that impair people's abilities to meet their most basic needs to the extent that they cause lasting harm or slow death (Farmer, 2010; Galtung, 1969). People in the camps experienced diminished independence and extremes of poverty. Accommodation was flimsy and crowded. Poor conditions led to disease (Finnström, 2008).

In an overview of NGO health interventions in the IDP camps, Dolan (2009) argues that

> the doctrine of minimal assistance ... went hand in hand with implicit criticism. People with no access to resources were told they were having sexual relations too young, not feeding their children a balanced diet, not planning their families well and having too many children they could not feed properly as a result. (p. 143)

This indictment of humanitarian interventions demonstrates how criticism of sexuality and childbearing practices prevailed alongside conditions that limited women's autonomy regarding both sex and family planning. In IDP camps, the unmet need for family planning was high, at 58 per cent in comparison to a national rate of about 40 per cent (Austin et al., 2008, p. 14). What Dolan refers to as an "implicit criticism" can also be understood as a health responsibilization message, based on ideals, here clearly misplaced, of individual choice and patient empowerment (Foley, 2008; Ruhl, 1999). This was particularly pernicious in a context in which people had limited control over the daily conditions in which they lived.

A UNICEF study of gender-based violence in Pabo IDP camp, nearby to Amuru, found that girls and women were "easily forced into marriage with men who [were] not of their choice, lured into sex for survival in the camp and above all lacking the power to negotiate for safe sex" (Akumu et al., 2005, p. 26). Sexual violence impacts women's reproductive health over their lifetime. As Westerhaus et al. (2007) describe:

> Women who tend crops and collect firewood on the perimeters of the camps are frequently attacked and raped by both Ugandan soldiers and members of the LRA. Additionally, women are frequently driven to transactional sex (i.e. providing sexual services for money) in order to provide for their children and attain the means to provide educational opportunities for their children. (p. 1184)

Women and girls in IDP camps experienced sexual violence with similar potential to impact their health and well-being as the violence recounted in the above discussion of abducted girls. For example, Patel et al. (2014b) find that "all young people in northern Ugandan have been similarly affected by HIV infection during war and displacement" (p. 1), making the case that the narrow focus on those who were abducted is counterproductive. Within the camps, "community mechanisms that would have protected girls [were] seriously limited in a context of eroded cultural and societal checks and balances" (Okello & Hovil, 2007, p. 441). This erosion contributed to the high incidence of sexual violence.

During lulls in fighting, some people commuted daily to their gardens to grow food, but many were often unable to tend their gardens. Instead, people in the camps relied on humanitarian assistance for food and feared rebel violence. They often stayed hidden in the days after a relief distribution, anticipating rebel raids (Finnström, 2008). The rebels, at times, tried to force people back home, exhorting them to leave and then burning the closely packed huts in the camp. Some people survived in the camps for over a decade in conditions that led Dolan (2009) to theorize that the camps were part of a strategy of social torture characterizing the conflict as a whole. Despite hardship and violence, as

Finnström (2008) argues, people were able to carve out limited space for personal agency in the camps. Life went on, but its daily patterns necessarily changed.

The process of return has been "complex, arduous and protracted" for those who were displaced (McElroy, 2012, p. 19). For people without a claim to land, there was no return option; they remained in or near the disbanded camps. Those returning home managed a life in two places at once as they worked to build homes, latrines, and bathing shelters and to clear, plough, and plant their land so that there would be a harvest. McElroy (2012) examines consequences for children's health resulting from how resettlement took place, with many problems she identifies, including poverty, food insecurity, and lack of access to health care and education, affecting the whole community. The challenges of return were ongoing and continued to affect people's lives as they worked to rebuild their communities.

### Ongoing Social Distress: Land Conflicts and Disease Epidemics

Beyond understanding this area as in recovery from conflict, it is important to recognize that regional disparities and divisions continue to cause distress today. My fieldwork took place in the year of the controversial KONY 2012 social media campaign that called for 2012 to be the year in which international forces collaborated to capture LRA leader Joseph Kony. Reactions to the campaign highlighted the need to shift the focus away from one notorious individual and towards current problems faced by many Acholi. The campaign, launched by the organization Invisible Children (IC, 2012), was criticized for its potential to hinder peace in the region through its call to arms and for the organization's remove from the local context, its failure to recognize local forms of justice, and other factors. For example, scholars who blogged on the campaign included Erin Baines (2012), who titled her piece "Ugandans 2012" and made the case that retribution was the wrong approach; Beth Stewart (2012), who wrote that targeting Kony would also mean targeting (abducted) children; and Akena Francis Adyanga (2012), who focused on problems of representation and characterized the campaign as exploitative. In the wake of this campaign, a neighbour (and health worker) remarked to me, "Joseph Kony could walk down Juba road today and nobody would see him," referring to a major route connecting to the south Sudanese capital. Amy Finnegan's (2013) critique of the IC campaign cites a reporter who finds that during rebuilding, "disease and land conflicts are the biggest problems – not Kony" (p. 31). The focus on capturing Kony indicates a disjuncture between

IC's assessment of the problem facing northern Uganda and local people's assessment. The latter pointed to disease, land conflicts, and lack of infrastructure. The controversy and anger surrounding the campaign highlights the potential for NGO-community tensions in the region, a theme of chapter 4.

While social media was drawing the West's attention to Kony, the immediate impact of disease epidemics and land grabs was more pressing to local residents than bringing down a villain. Local people celebrated an end to armed conflict, to be sure, yet for many, the threat of disease and ongoing uncertainty due to land issues meant that life could not return to normal. Agriculture was an ongoing way of life and yet poverty, accompanied by lack of access to resources, was a prominent feature of life for many in the area. In post-conflict northern Uganda, distressing and quotidian aspects of life exist side by side and contemporaneously.

### The Outbreak of Disease

Along with other common illnesses and poor access to basic health care, people in northern Uganda had to worry about the return of Ebola and about nodding disease. Nodding disease, which emerged in northern Uganda in 2007 after first being documented in southern Sudan in the 1990s, is an illness of unknown etiology that causes debilitating illness and death among children. Gulu was the epicentre of a major Ebola outbreak in late 2000 through early 2001 (Finnström, 2008; WHO, 2012) that eventually killed 224 people in three districts (Kinsman, 2012). Towards the end of my fieldwork period, in August 2012, a smaller outbreak of Ebola elsewhere in Uganda was a source of fear (the WHO reported 17 dead by the time the outbreak ended). I wrote in my field notes that I was obsessively reading news of the outbreak and noted, "In Kibaale, the only patients remaining in hospital are in the maternity ward. I was thinking that if this place [the health centre] had to shut down for quarantine, there would be nowhere for people to deliver." Amid the outbreak, people spoke to me about their experiences during the 2000–1 outbreak, remembering those who had suffered or died. Among those lost was Dr. Matthew Lukwiya (Figure 2.1), the supervising doctor at Lacor Hospital, who died while caring for patients in 2000 and is remembered for his courage and leadership (Coulter, 2001; Englert et al., 2018; Kinsman, 2012; Lacor Hospital, n.d.-b).

Anger over injustices in the country's north is evident when people speculate about the possible cause of nodding disease. Several thousand children in northern Uganda are suffering from this progressive and fatal illness, which is characterized by a nodding seizure that often

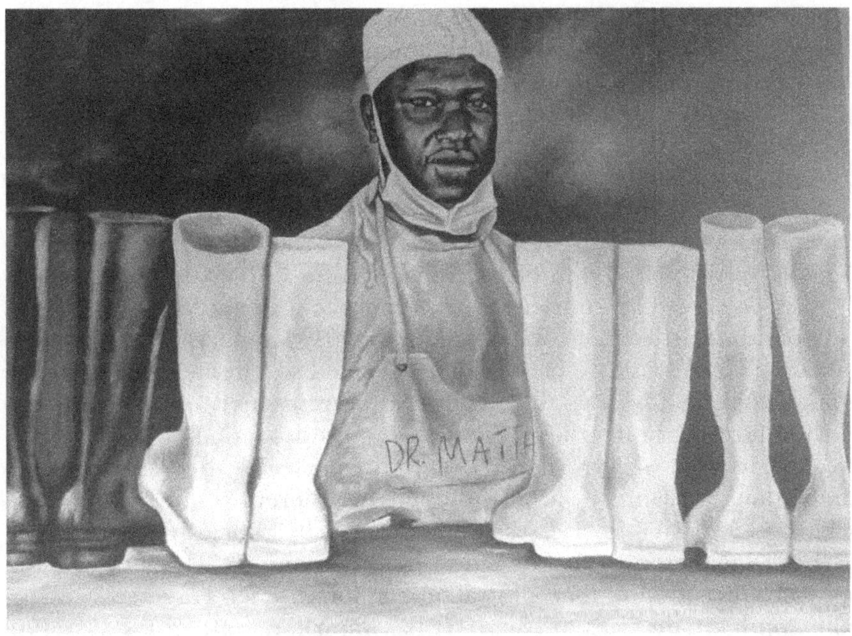


Figure 2.1.  Dr. Matthew, by Thomas Vava. (Used with the permission of the artist.)

manifests when food is presented (Lacey, 2003; Mitchell et al., 2013). Community members connected this new disease to the war:

> Despite the medical theories regarding potential causal agents in the etiology of nodding syndrome, the communities of Kitgum, Lamwo, and Pader strongly associate the temporal relationship of the war with the onset of nodding syndrome in their children. The LWF field officer assigned to address the impact of nodding syndrome in northern Uganda explains that, "Conclusively, people [in northern Uganda communities] say that this is a result of the war. Before the camps, there was no nodding syndrome." (Mitchell et al., 2013, p. 23)

Mitchell and colleagues cite beliefs among Acholi people that food aid or black fly were the cause of this devastating illness, while some Acholi members of parliament suggested a link to "atomic weapons" or poisoned food aid ("Acholi MPs Link Nodding Disease," 2012). Such rumours and misinformation about the causes of ill health proliferate during wartime. In a 2012 speech on peacebuilding in Gulu, Branch (2012) asked the following rhetorical question: "Perhaps bullets aren't being fired, but is Nodding Disease any less deadly?" summing up the anger over the perceived connection between war and the illness.

The stories surrounding nodding disease piqued my interest in health-related rumours. Finnström (2008) suggests that the literal truth of various disease-related rumours that circulated during the war is less important than the moral truth expressed by believing in or repeating such rumours. An example he cites of such a rumour was that the cooking oil provided in the internal displacement camps caused impotence. Finnström identifies rumours as an attempt to gain control over difficult surroundings. Like Finnström, Branch (2011) suggests that rumours about aid and health – such as that poisoned sorghum was responsible for a cholera outbreak – were significant as resistance to the larger context of forced displacement. With the camps disbanded, I observed that regarding disease outbreak and health care provision, the "bad surroundings" that gave Finnström his title persist, inherent in these unpredictable and untreatable diseases and in the paucity of health care services.

High incidence of HIV infection has been one challenge during the post-conflict context. The clinical officer, Jonas, when I asked him about the approximate rates at Lacor HCIII, Amuru, described the HIV rate among pregnant couples as follows: "Every day you test people, if you test thirty you will find at least three, three here [who are HIV positive]," approximately reflecting reported rates in the region, discussed in further detail in chapter 5.

In addition to fear of disease, access to basic health care remains an ongoing struggle. Providing health care, or failing to provide health care, can have an important symbolic and pragmatic value, in that it can be interpreted to signal the ill or good will of the government towards the north and the inclusion or exclusion of northern Uganda by the government. As well as affecting health, the way health care is provided or withheld provides messages about citizenship (Sinding, 2010, p. 1657). Shortages of staff, medication, supplies, and facilities exist throughout Uganda but were particularly prominent in the north, where the building of infrastructure postwar has been slow. The failure to meet government standards for health centre distribution means that for most people, access to basic health care is challenging and contributes to ongoing social distress post-conflict. The difficulty of access to health care particularly affected pregnant women, who were expected to attend a health centre for four antenatal appointments and for delivery, despite lack of health centre coverage and other access barriers (detailed in chapter 3). In a piece examining the benefits and pitfalls of truth and reconciliation processes, the Acholi poet and scholar Juliane Okot Bitek (2012) shows that nodding disease, the violence of war, and the violence of poverty are inseparable, suggesting too that the spiritual impacts and physical impacts of the conflict are inherent in each other:

> The *cen* are here.
>
> What more physical manifestations do you need after you've stumbled on random tibiae and femurs and tripped over skulls, still toothed, in open grassy fields?
>
> What more physical manifestations do you need all these years after the war, and bombs lie waiting, only to detonate when kin, or neighbours, or people you don't even know are blown up on a regular enough basis and that only deserves a shrug from others who hear of it?
>
> What more physical manifestations do you need than heaps and heaps of stones waiting to be crushed by women, men, children who should be in school but can't because the whole family has to be employed, or nobody has dinner?
>
> What more physical manifestations do you need?
>
> The *cen* are in your dreams, a lot, not every day.
>
> The *cen* are in the neighbour's child, now seized by epileptic fits since the daughter returned from the bush. Who knows what she did over there to whom?
>
> The *cen* are now in the constant nodding of children being harvested in the hundreds. (p. 394)

In Okot Bitek's poem, *cen* manifest around unburied remains, land mines, abject labour, and nodding disease. Each of these is a feature of the post-conflict context. The health consequences of conflict, displacement, and post-conflict cannot be separated from the social and political consequences.

### Agriculture

Among the losses of war were many related to agriculture. Absence from land because of abduction or internment, the destruction of trees and crops, and the theft of livestock had a devastating and in some cases lasting impact. The chief local economic activity, subsistence agriculture, returned, not unchanged, but enough to dominate social and economic life. While money and paid work were hard to come by, work itself was not. The majority of adults and older children grew food for their families and for sale in local markets. They worked in their fields and gardens, ploughing, planting, and harvesting with hand tools. After food was harvested, much of it needed to be dried and pounded before consumption. Most Acholi in Amuru lived, after they had dispersed from the camps, in small and often remote household settings. This tie to the land contributed to the difficulties of transportation (discussed in chapter 3), since even as improvements were made to main roads, many people still lived in unfrequented areas. The wartime theft of cattle and destruction of mango trees, and the need to reclaim fields, paths, and waterways that had overgrown in the years of displacement, had limited the scope of agriculture. This loss of the everyday activities of farming, and the inability to pass related skills and traditions to youth, loomed large among returnees (Gauvin, 2013). While the war interrupted economic life, the work of farming was something people could return to, a well-known rhythm giving shape to the calendar year and sustenance for life.

Women have been responsible for a large portion of this rebuilding work (Oosterom, 2011). The increased workload has persisted since the time of the camps, when gender roles shifted such that women shouldered additional responsibilities:

> Women indicated it is they who bring up and "teach" the children, and do the bulk of the household work, as well as most cultivation. Even though men can be seen working in the gardens, digging in groups or with the ox-plough, it is, according to the women, done less than before the camp."
> (Oosterom, 2011, p. 404)

For many women, the need to undertake heavy work was a challenge to ensuring a healthy pregnancy, as I discuss in chapter 3. This could be shaped by male partners' willingness or unwillingness to share the workload during pregnancy. Increased alcohol use among men, a problem in the camps and in the post-conflict period (Annan & Brier, 2010; Oosterom, 2011), had affected some men's willingness or ability to be supportive during pregnancy.

Material impacts include the land disputes and poverty described in this chapter. There were no questions in my interview script, which mostly focused on pregnancy and care, about land disputes, but several participants brought up the issue. Anita was someone who had been particularly impacted, because her husband was imprisoned over such a dispute and was not present to support her during pregnancy. A 20-year-old mother of two, she was pregnant with their third and worried about money. At first, I found it contradictory that she said he had been jailed for a land dispute and then said he had been poaching; I felt perhaps her first explanation was an attempt to save face. Only as I learned more about land disputes did I realize that criminalizing and policing as "poaching" what would formerly have been hunting was a way of pushing people off land and a denial of their previously undisputed rights. Land disputes and related evictions and imprisonment are an example of ongoing social distress after the end to the LRA conflict. Focus group participants in Lujoro referred to the loss of "wealth that walks on its legs," particularly cattle and goats, as a significant impact that the conflict had on people's ability to be healthy. The impacts of the post-conflict setting and ongoing social distress varied greatly between individual study participants, but taken collectively, their experiences indicate that these contexts are important to the social coordination of maternity care and birth.

### Land Disputes

Because of the economic dependency on agriculture and to the social significance of land as a site of paternal lineage, "to lose their land is perhaps what Acholi people fear most" (Finnström, 2008, p. 179). In the context of returnees negotiating relationships to paternal clans, Baines explains that "land is a sign of rootedness, connectedness, and belonging in Acholi, where farming and garden work are processes of building social relatedness and ties within the clan" (in Amony, 2015, p. 149). Land disputes also greatly complicated the work required by returnees who relied on farming for food and income generation. These disputes have occurred both between local families, and between residents and outside interests such as government initiatives or corporate sugarcane farmers. In a "judicial vacuum" (Finnström, 2008, p. 179) in which land tenure has not generally been identified through legal title but instead through less formal processes such as passing gardens down through generations, disagreements over land disputes can be difficult to resolve and have led to violence.

Individual or family disputes over who owns or has the right to farm land have arisen because of the long years spent in IDP camps, away from the fields. Although many still visited their gardens, some gardens were too far or too dangerous and thus lay fallow. Disputes among individuals or families have been a complication of resettlement, as some people returned to their place only to be pushed out (observation and personal communication with Jonas; "Uganda: Land Disputes," 2012).

On a larger scale, land disputes have arisen because of government and corporate takeovers of traditional Acholi lands. In Apaa, located on a contested boundary between Amuru district and Adjumani district in the West Nile area, there is an ongoing land dispute. One dimension is disagreement over whether land was part of a wildlife reserve, as the Uganda Wildlife Authority claims, or was the customary land of its residents. This dispute, which has been characterized as a "green land grab" (Serwajja, 2018) has led to forced evictions, violence between neighbouring villages, and decreased food production capacity (Refugee Law Project, 2012). In 2012, one man was killed in a police eviction from this land (Webb, 2012); 2018 saw renewed hut burnings, evictions, and deaths (Laing & Weschler, 2018). In May 2018, the Acholi cultural leader and others released a statement condemning human rights violations and land seizure in Apaa; in an unprecedented civic action in July 2018, Apaa residents encamped themselves at the Gulu offices of the United Nations Office of the High Commissioner for Human Rights in a protest that Laing and Weschler (2018) have referred to as a chosen displacement. Experienced with the exigencies of camp life, the protesters "established joint daily rhythms of strategy meetings and prayers, and created groups responsible for overseeing medical care, song-writing, games and practical tasks" (Laing & Weschler, 2018, para. 10). In 2012, the potential for land to be appropriated for the Apaa wildlife reserve was a concern among residents in Teddi, one of the six villages where I interviewed childbearing women (personal communication with local leader, Teddi, July 3, 2012); at the time of writing, this dispute remains ongoing.

In addition to the dispute over wildlife reserve boundaries, corporate interests were taking over "unused land" for large-scale agriculture and production; in Amuru, the Madhvani group was involved in disputed land for its sugar cane production (Barnabas, 2013; Owor & Dieterle, 2020). This led to situations in which corporate representatives said the land was populated only by squirrels, while local women protested by stripping down, a form of protest and shaming (Lawino, 2012). Barnabas (2013) sums up the complexity of land disputes as follows:

> The dynamics of land conflicts in Northern Uganda is linked to the historical legacy of the Lord's Resistance Army (LRA) rebellion and the consequential displacement, return and resettlement and population settlement, weak land administration and governance, politics and investment, mineral wealth and curses, creation of new districts and individual greed to mention but a few. (p. 018)

Since farming and other land-based economic activities, such as beekeeping or collecting wood for charcoal, made up both a livelihood and a life for the majority of people in this area, disputes over land tenure have had a significant impact on individuals and communities. As Branch (2011) writes:

> Acholiland perhaps is being reconstructed, but various forms of violence and exclusion continue within Acholi society, particularly around contestations over land and political authority, and continue to characterize the

relation between the Acholi and the national government – the very conditions that gave rise to the rebellions and then sustained them for over twenty years. (p. 10)

Just as the decades of conflict and displacement have shaped the overall social landscape in which maternity care and birth take place, so too have disputes over land tenure and the outbreaks of diseases. This is the case when land disputes or illness affected the families of childbearing women, as well as in how such features of ongoing social distress have impacted the broader social well-being of people in this area. The impact of land disputes varied from village to village and contributed to my decision to include several villages in the study.

### Poverty and Lack of Infrastructure

Widespread poverty and an accompanying lack of infrastructure affected people's day-to-day lives. Poverty and lack of infrastructure have been shaped by the past conflict but were far from unique to this region or setting. While some aspects of community life, such as gardening and house building, followed generations-old practices, this way of life had also been overlaid with a capitalist economy and its demands. From school fees to airtime for mobile phones, there was a need for money that, for most people, was hard to meet via the income generated by selling food surpluses or other small-scale income-generation activities. A lack of infrastructure further compounded the effects of poverty. Poor roads contributed to the difficulty, cost, and danger of transportation; a paucity of operational health facilities made health services less accessible and more costly in time and money; and the list went on. Maternity care and birth, alongside other aspects of life, were affected by a lack of money and infrastructure. Taken together, these insufficiencies are a form of structural violence.

### Impacts on Study Participants' Experiences of Pregnancy and Birth

In each village where we interviewed women, I asked Acero to share her impressions and recorded notes about distinguishing features such as the presence or absence of livestock, beehives, and household gardens; whether school-aged children were at home or in school; and path/road conditions. Local leaders, who we met with at the outset and conclusion of our time in their village, shared their concerns regarding issues facing their community, in relation to pregnancy and birth and more generally. They brought up concerns such as land seizure and lack of school facilities (Teddi), HIV (Rec Kicere), and alcohol abuse and relationship breakdown (Turdakatuba). Leaders understood these broader social concerns, many of which are discussed above, as important to women's health. Participants described some of their experiences during the conflict as they told me about their approaches to pregnancy, care, and birth. The conflict shaped participants' experiences in physical, spiritual, social, and material ways. Taken together, these stories illustrate how the conflict and the post-conflict setting influenced how women approached maternity care and birth.

Physical repercussions of the conflict included injuries that affected reproductive well-being. For example, Faith worried during pregnancy because of an injury she had received as a child, during her abduction by the LRA. She had been shot in the side of her abdomen, an injury to which she attributed a previous miscarriage. A 24-year-old mother of four, she reported that as well as being painful because of her injury, pregnancy was a distressing time as she worried that she might miscarry again. Another woman from the same village, Mildred, had burns to her ribcage and upper thigh incurred during the conflict. They made pregnancy uncomfortable for her, but she was able to safely deliver healthy children – she had five. Their neighbour, Betty, asked if it was okay for her to speak about her husband. He had been beaten with a machete across his back and neck and left for dead during the war. Betty told us that he had since been advised by doctors not to work or ride a bicycle. However, with 10 children to raise, some of whom were born to a deceased relative, both he and Betty found it impossible to take the rest that health care workers advised. The conversations about war injuries were difficult for participants to share and were hard to hear, but participants felt they were important to discuss. The physical injuries remaining from the war impacted the physical experience of pregnancy, as well as adding to the emotional and material challenges.

The spiritual impacts of war speak to ongoing psychosocial trauma caused by loss and witnessing or experiencing violence. Janice told me that during two of her pregnancies, a bad spirit (*cen*) would come to her in quiet moments and speak to her. She recalled the *cen* telling her "Janice, you are going to die in childbirth." Janice attributed this encounter to the many who had been killed nearby and whose remains had been allowed to go unburied for some time. Her home was in an area that was known as having been hit particularly hard during the war; when driving near that area with health centre staff, they shared stories of wartime atrocities. As in most cultures, the burial of the dead is significant to Acholi people. Amony and Baines (Amony 2015, p. 152) identify a widespread concern that those who were left unburied might have their remains eaten by animals and never be at rest. After being prayed for by born-again Christians, Janice told me, she was free from spirits in a subsequent pregnancy. Baines (2017) explores life narratives and demonstrates how "for a woman in a subordinate and vulnerable position, spirit possession can be a mechanism through which it is possible to call attention to harm endured, and to seek redress" (p. 107). However one interprets it, the story of the *cen* with a message of death during birth was significant to Janice.

For Florence, a focus group participant, the spiritual impact of war might also be understood as a loss of mental health, which she had since recovered. She said that after seeing a ghost of a man who looked like her brother-in-law (who was still living) several times, she found herself going from shop to shop begging for candy, without realizing what she was doing. In the same focus group, participants shared stories of spirits that would strangle a pregnant woman during birth; the remedy was to have a witch doctor provide a cleansing. Participants shared stories that attributed the deaths of one woman in labour and one child to such a strangling spirit. Spiritual explanations for "misfortune and ill-health" have a long history in Acholi cosmology (P'Bitek, 1971, p. 160). The inherent uncertainties and worries of pregnancy were underscored by spiritual impacts arising from the past conflict. These physical and spiritual injuries are ones that participants offered as having a direct connection to their war years. The overall social world of maternity care in Amuru, which I continue to explore in the next chapters, has also been influenced by the past conflict, albeit in ways that are difficult to separate from other social and institutional factors.

## Conclusion

War and other complex humanitarian emergencies necessarily impact maternal mortality and other aspects of maternal-child health (Austin et al., 2008). Sub-Saharan African countries that have experienced recent armed conflict have significantly higher rates of maternal mortality than those that have not, and also have lower skilled attendance at deliveries (O'Hare & Southall, 2007, p. 565). Women and health workers in northern Uganda during the post-conflict period worried about deaths during childbirth as well as other poor outcomes (Chi et al., 2015a). Conflict and recent conflict, then, are significant in shaping experiences and outcomes of pregnancy and care. The structural, social, and individual harms arising from conflict are highly relevant to how maternity care and birth are socially organized in Amuru sub-county, northern Uganda.

Working with IE, it was important for me to "learn about the material features of the economic, historical, political, and social contexts in which people's lives occur. Within these are clues about the social and ruling relations organizing people's social experience" (Bisaillon, 2012, p. 609). In Amuru, a return to "normal" – to agriculture, to living with family, to relying on long-established social supports – exists in tandem with social distress resulting from the traumas of the conflict, as well as from ongoing sites of struggle for rights and citizenship, including health and land tenure. This social context affects how maternity care and birth are organized. The setting I have described here informs my analysis in the upcoming chapters. It impacts health care provision and the effect of lack of resources, discussed in chapter 3; it impacts the role of the basic goods that NGOs provide to mothers, discussed in chapter 4, and it impacts the interplay between power, gender, and HIV testing during ANC, discussed in chapter 5.

# Chapter Three

# Pregnancy and Daily Life: Health System and Home Factors Shaping Care

## Introduction

Approaches to care and birth in Amuru, northern Uganda, are structured by everyday challenges associated with poverty and lack of infrastructure. Among these, accessing transportation, avoiding arduous physical work while pregnant, and ensuring adequate nutrition are pervasive. In this chapter, I provide a snapshot of how and by whom ANC and maternity care services were offered in Amuru sub-county. I also map the social landscape for maternity care, with a focus on transportation, nutrition, and work as factors coordinating the social context of maternity care.

## Focused (Goal-Oriented) Antenatal Care

Throughout Uganda, focused ANC, also referred to as *goal-oriented ANC*, is offered. This approach is intended to achieve specific outcomes in a small number of visits. Focused ANC is a departure from a risk-based approach, familiar in the global north, which classifies pregnant women as high or low risk over many ANC visits throughout pregnancy (Lincetto et al., 2006, p. 53). It is argued that a weakness of a risk-based approach is that many women designated high-risk do not develop complications, while others identified as low risk do develop complications (Lincetto et al., 2006). Attending a large number of appointments is not feasible for many pregnant women in the global south for whom transportation challenges and other costs associated with ANC pose barriers; a focused approach addresses this challenge (Lincetto et al., 2006). Focused ANC is intended to reduce the high cost to health care systems and individuals that are associated with a risk-based approach that includes more visits. The WHO has adopted focused ANC consisting of four, later revised to eight, visits and specified activities as its recommended practice (Conrad et al., 2012, p. 301).

Uganda's 2016 clinical guidelines (UMOH, 2016) identify the goals of ANC, to be met over four ANC appointments, as follows:

> Prevention and treatment of any complications; Emergency preparedness; Birth planning; Satisfying any unmet nutritional, social, emotional and physical needs of the pregnant woman; Provision of patient education, including successful care and nutrition of the newborn; Identification of high-risk pregnancy; Encouragement of (male) partner involvement in antenatal care.

While Uganda's 2016 clinical guidelines continued to specify four visits, on a 2019 visit to Lacor and Amuru, I learned that women were being encouraged to go to the health centre for ANC eight times or once a month, but that late first appointments, occurring after the first trimester, made this difficult (personal communication, Christophe, April 24, 2019; personal communication, E. Ochola, April 25, 2019). This change is in accordance with the WHO guidelines introduced in 2016, with the hope that an increase in contact with health providers would improve outcomes (WHO, 2016).

Florence, a focus group participant, described her experience of ANC as follows:

> When I entered the health centre, the health worker welcomed me. I was examined and found that the person inside my stomach was fine. I was given medicine and told to continue with the check-ups and the good health. If I felt any pain then I should move with my card [i.e., take the ANC card to the health centre] and get medicine for that part that is paining. So I continued to protect that pregnancy and completed the check-ups up to the time of delivery.

She focused on the role of ANC in ensuring the health of the baby and in protecting the pregnancy. Her description suggests a participatory role in managing her health and health care during pregnancy. Most ANC visits took place as she describes, at the health centre. On outreach visits to remote areas for another purpose, such as immunization, midwives were present and available to examine pregnant women, but outreach visits to any given community were infrequent, and patients were generally required to travel to a health centre to receive ANC.

Another important feature of ANC as it was provided in Amuru was the ANC card mentioned by Florence. Issued to women at their first appointment, this card recorded women's health information as pertinent to pregnancy, including their age, the number and outcome of previous pregnancies, and their HIV status. Women were required to keep their card and to show it at health centre visits, including at the time of delivery. Participants sometimes saw ANC attendance and the ANC card as a key to making health centre delivery possible, referring to ANC as "catching the card," a dynamic I explore in chapter 4. Throughout Uganda, HIV testing for pregnant women and their partners (couples' testing) was also offered, ideally in the first antenatal visit, a site of complexity that I examine in chapter 5.

## The Message to Attend ANC

Despite all the challenges to reaching care, I found that overwhelmingly, the participants with whom I spoke were familiar with the public health message to attend ANC. Health care workers conveyed the importance of attending ANC during their outreach visits to villages, the primary purpose of which was immunization and that also included mobile ANC. This message was also disseminated through signs near the health centre, as in Figure 3.1; at group public health talks held at the health centre while patients were waiting for care;[1] through the work of the VHT and among them the TBAs; and through radio announcements.

Each of these forms of messaging had its respective advantages and drawbacks: some women indicated that they never listened to the radio, while others told me that outreach had not reached their village. The women I spoke with all had attended at least one appointment, demonstrating that the message to attend ANC was at least partially successful. This was consistent with national trends: in Uganda, 94 per cent of rural women attended ANC for at least one visit in 2011, while by 2016, there was a reported national upswing in the percentage of women attending four or more visits to about 60 per cent, from 48 per cent in 2011. Rurality, poverty, and low level of educational attainment all decreased the likelihood that a woman would report having received skilled health care (Uganda Bureau of Statistics, 2011, 2016). These numbers make it clear that ANC is a known service; however, lower rates of women attending a full complement of ANC (four

---

1 Health talks or health education referred to information shared by health workers with groups of people who were gathered waiting for care in the reception area of the health centre or who had gathered at a central place near their home to receive outreach. Lacor Health Centre III Amuru employed a public health educator who was responsible for such programming. Other health workers also gave talks on topics including hygiene and other public health issues.

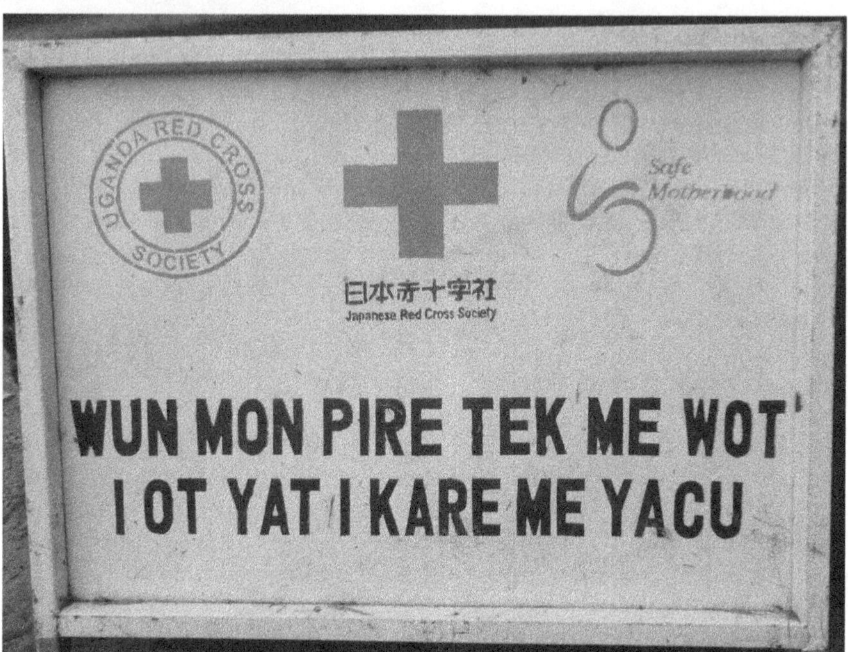


Figure 3.1. Sign on visiting the health centre. The English translation is "Women: It is important to come to the hospital/health centre when you are pregnant." The supporting agencies are represented in English and Japanese with their logos. (Source: Sarah Rudrum.)

appointments) indicate ongoing challenges, as does the fact that delivery care rates continue to lag behind ANC rates. Since most maternal deaths occur in proximity to delivery, skilled delivery care is the more important indicator for improved outcomes. In Uganda overall, birth at a facility rose from 57 per cent reported in 2011 to 73 per cent in 2016 for births occurring in the five years before the survey (Uganda Bureau of Statistics, 2011; 2016). In addition to health messaging, the practice of giving a mama kit at the time of delivery was seen by both childbearing women and health workers as a way to reinforce the message to use formal health services, a practice I further examine in chapter 4.

While childbearing women knew that ANC attendance was highly encouraged, the reason for going (i.e., optimal health) was not always understood in the same way by pregnant patients as by health workers. Participants often referred to attending ANC as "catching the card," emphasizing receiving the ANC card as an important aspect of ANC participation. After speaking to a number of mothers, I came to recognize that the ANC card acted as a ticket or key to access health services. For example, Anita, a 20-year-old mother of two, described ANC attendance as like "a key, because when you reach the hospital like this then you hand in your [ANC] card and they see how many times this person has tested, what problems have been got." ANC and the ANC card, from women's perspectives, acted as a means to coordinating care at the time of labour. While women recognized the health benefits of ANC, women also attended ANC because they felt they must. Faith, who had been abducted and shot in the abdomen during the LRA/UNPDF conflict and worried about miscarriage resulting from her old injury, said that ANC attendance had been described to her as akin to a "law." In her account, ANC is closely linked to testing for HIV, referred to here as *sickness*:

> So they [VHT or outreach health workers] say when you are pregnant it is like a law: you have to go to the hospital for ANC so that you understand how your health is. If they find that you have sickness they guide you on how you should live, so that they help the child you are carrying in your womb.

Attending ANC was viewed as complying with a law or obtaining a key, as well as supporting a healthy pregnancy and delivery.

**The Provision of Mama Kits**

In Amuru, an NGO project distributed mama kits, a bag containing baby basics: soap, a washing basin, towels, jelly (baby cream), and sheets, towels, or cloths (for tying the baby to the mother's back, for warmth, for drying, and to absorb blood). The kits offset expenses of about US$5, a significant amount of money in this low-income context (Mbonye et al., 2013, p. 5). They also contained items to be used by health centre staff, including tetracycline eye ointment (to prevent or treat neonatal eye infections). The mama kits were given to women by health centre staff at the time of birth in the health centre and were a project of the Red Cross. Women who wanted to receive one were required to register with, and receive a registration card from, their local VHT member. Registration took place via outreach in pregnant women's home villages or on a given day at the health centre. In practice, registration and distribution was a complex process involving multiple stakeholders and impacting how women approached care. Distribution was not universal; not every mother received a kit after giving birth. In the context of poverty, the past conflict, and parallel ongoing NGO involvement and NGO withdrawal, material resources acted to shape childbearing women's experiences and practices. In chapter 4, I further identify how the mama kits project was a site that concentrated the operation of power and affected access to care.

## Formal Health Care Providers

### *The Setting for Formal Health Care Provision*

Throughout Uganda, NGO-run health centres and hospitals operate alongside government-run facilities, supplementing the health system to make up for the gap in capacity and quality at state-run facilities. Private, for-profit facilities are also part of this mix, but are mainly centred in the capital, Kampala, and its surrounds (United States Agency for International Development [USAID], 2015). In Amuru, most maternity care was provided at the health centre, a series of wards and offices joined by open air corridors and located in a gated compound at the site of a former IDP camp. This health centre was one of three rural HCIIIs operated by a Canadian and Italian Catholic non-profit organization as an offshoot of a major hospital, Saint Mary's Lacor (very near Gulu town, in Lacor). Lacor hospital is widely regarded as offering exemplary care, as is the case for its rural health centres, and is a hospital with deep connections to people and place. The story goes that the health centre in Amuru opened after one of the hospital's founding doctors, Dr. Corti, was gored by a water buffalo and badly injured while visiting the area, leading him to observe the lack of health care facilities where sick or injured people in this remote area could seek treatment. This was the spark behind the founding of the health centre in the mid-1970s, which the Italian doctor opened alongside his Canadian wife, Dr. Lucille Teasdale-Corti, and they together operated Lacor Hospital. Dr. Teasdale-Corti, who died of professionally acquired HIV/AIDS and is buried alongside her husband at the hospital, was a recipient of the Order of Canada and the subject of a 2004 heritage minute (Cowley, 2013). Their daughter, Dr. Dominque Corti, continues to play a leadership role at the hospital.

Despite the international ties of Lacor, all staff at the rural health centre were Acholi (visiting and expatriate international health workers, including doctors and pharmacists, contributed to the staffing of the main hospital site). Health centre staff also made periodic outreach trips to remote areas of the sub-county, outreach that included vaccinations, health talks, and antenatal check-ups. I observed some ANC examinations that took place roadside in the shade and privacy of the ambulance. However, there were barriers to relying on outreach for ANC. At an antenatal visit, women would be given a date by which to come for their next appointment. They would be fined if they missed that date (interview with Jacky). Outreach trips occurred relatively infrequently, meaning that women could not rely on outreach to provide the required number of ANC visits.

In contrast to studies documenting a tense or disrespectful relationship between health care workers and their patients in Uganda, even extending to the abuse of pregnant women (Amooti-Kaguna & Nuwaha, 2000; Kyomuhendo, 2003), most participants described an overall positive relation to caregivers at the health centre. This corroborated my own impression of a professional warmth in the quality of care. For example, Erin, who wore a "get rid of neglected diseases for better health" T-shirt during her interview, had to transfer to the hospital for her most recent delivery and mentioned the warm reception at the health centre and the quick response to emergencies as something that should continue, when I asked her to suggest recommendations for change. Grace alluded to a narrative that health workers fostered bad relations with their patients, emphasizing that this was not her own experience. She told me, "You know, in the village, they say that the nurses do not help people, they only make fun of you. But when I reached the hospital, I saw them welcome me well. There was no fun made on me." Lily was also happy with her reception but framed a warm welcome as provisional, saying, "They welcomed me well because I had my [ANC] card." A positive reception of patients was important to the women I spoke with and indeed is a necessary feature of quality health care.

While one of the TBAs mentioned that having only bad or ripped clothes could be a reason mothers avoided care, a comment supported by the literature, there was no other evidence of this type of practice within my research. One of the nursing staff, when I asked how she would respond to a patient who had no clean cloth with her to wrap the newborn baby, told me she would bring a *kitenge* from her room and give it to the patient. I wrote in my field notes about the daily lives of health workers and their similarity to those of patients, despite the disparity in educational attainment and status: "The health workers here, without exception, also have land that they are farming or having farmed by others. Almost all have children. The children are sometimes out of school because of no school fees or no money for school uniforms. As well as farming, the food prep is intense: people buy or grow cassava, cut it, dry it, and pound or peel it to make *posho* or pancakes. They grow (or buy) then shell, roast, and pound groundnuts and *simsim* [sesame seeds], then make them into sauces or snacks. They raise and kill chickens ... As much as there is sometimes a real and perceived class/education/economic divide between health workers and their patients, many of their lifeways, much of their work, is similar." These similarities were particularly prominent with lower-status health workers.

Importantly, all of the health workers shared an ethnicity and mother tongue with their patients, which is not always the case in African settings where there is great cultural diversity and inequities in education and career expectations. In my observation, health workers approached their role with professionalism, with some reporting it as a calling. Frustrations did exist towards patients. Gloria mentioned having to report the deaths of mothers who ignore referral to hospital as one source of difficulty at work. She told me, "When you lose a mother, it's so painful. Writing 'what what,' despite the fact that I've referred … but when we have maternal death, I need to report. So it's painful, though due to her, this state." It was clear that in addition to the pain over the mother's death, she faced an additional burden of responsibility, even when, in her assessment, the patient's failure to follow the referral to a hospital is to blame. Overall, the potential for poor relations was something participants were aware of while mainly describing their interactions in positive ways that indicated mutual respect and care.

Several participants,[2] however, mentioned that they gave birth unattended by a care provider at the health centre. When I followed up with health workers and administrators, they attributed this partly to the fact that, at night, patients sometimes bypassed the room where they should have checked in and went directly to the staff housing area above the health centre proper, thus delaying access to care. I witnessed this happen in the case of a motorcycle accident at night: seeing the health centre mostly dark and lights on at my home, the victim's friend came to my door to ask for help. My field notes record, "J. said he stitched him ear to ear. A few days later, he came back: the wound was septic, and J. had to re-do it." Understaffing was also a factor in contributing to unattended births at the health centre, based on the accounts of those who had given birth unattended, as well as Jonas's description. Despite some shortcomings, Lacor HCIII Amuru met the conditions for skilled attendance, especially when contrasted to the available government-run health care services.

*Clinical Officers*

Within Amuru sub-county, there were no doctors participating in care to pregnant and birthing women. Amuru district had only one HCIV, which was required to have a doctor; it was located in Atiak, a town north of Amuru sub-county near the border with South Sudan. The most senior

---

2 Specifically, Sara and Amelia from Rec Kicere, Penny from Oberabic, and Rose from Turdakatuba.

health care worker required at any HCIII is a clinical officer. Throughout sub-Saharan Africa, particularly in rural areas, clinical officers fill the gap left by the shortage of doctors: "Clinical officers have a separate training from medical doctors, but their roles include many medical and surgical tasks usually carried out by doctors" (Wilson et al., 2011, para. 3). A benefit of the clinical officer program is that there is a diminished risk of brain drain; qualified physicians have greater international mobility than clinical officers. There was one clinical officer at Lacor HCIII Amuru, Jonas (a study participant). He split his role between clinical and senior administrative work, and the midwives and nursing staff members reported to him. While he would attend a birth if other staff members were unavailable, he did not work scheduled shifts in the labour ward or antenatal clinic.

*Midwives*

At the time of my fieldwork, two midwives were employed at Lacor HCIII. This was in keeping with recommended numbers. The roadmap on maternal health states that "according to the current staffing norms, HCIIIs and HCIVs are provided with 2 and 4 midwives respectively but these are inadequate, besides the fact that many positions are not filled. There is inequitable distribution of personnel between districts and between urban and rural settings" (UMOH, 2006, p. 11). The problem of understaffing of midwives was observable in the sub-county, with other health centres in the sub-county employing a single midwife or no midwife. For example, a health centre in Oberabic serving a large parish (Acwera) had, in mid-2012, hired its first midwife. In Uganda, midwives are formally trained, with three years of postsecondary education, and are registered with the Midwifery Council. Their work centres on antenatal, delivery, and post-partum care. Midwives also participate in outreach trips and provide mobile ANC services. Nurses had a broader range of responsibilities than midwives, including work in other wards, but also participated in maternity care, as detailed next.

*Enrolled Comprehensive Nurses, Registered Nurses,*
*Nursing Assistants, and Nurse Aides*

In addition to midwives, a range of nursing staff members provided care to pregnant and birthing women. The qualifications of nursing staff varied significantly. The most senior were enrolled comprehensive nurses (ECNs), who are comprehensive nurses who hold a certificate and have additional midwifery training and are enrolled with the Nurse's Council. Registered nurses (RNs) hold diplomas in general nursing. In contrast to these formally trained and accredited nurses, nursing assistants and particularly nurse aides at the health centre had little formal training. Nursing assistants had between three months and one year of classroom training, focusing on basic patient care. Nurse aides had no classroom training; they were trained on the job. Their duties included cleaning and patient care. At Lacor HCIII, nurse aides were hired from local communities (interview with Jonas; Matsiko & Kiwanuka, 2003). Some nurse aides were selected to undertake further training to become nursing assistants. Lacor HCIII employed one ECN, one RN, several nursing assistants, and several nurse aides. While only an ECN has equivalent maternity care skills and training to a midwife (interview with Jonas), all levels of nursing staff, including nurse aides who were laypeople, attended deliveries. Due to minimal staffing, scheduling for double coverage of health workers on the delivery ward was not always possible; staff members often worked alone, particularly at night. Women who gave birth at the health centre, then, received care from practitioners with a wide range of skill-levels and training, from laypeople to highly trained professionals. This complicates the assumption that giving birth at a health centre means receiving care from a SBA. Occasionally, as mentioned, women gave birth at the health centre unattended.

Early on at the health centre, while I was still working to understand people's roles and positions, I wrote about basic health care for the children of the health centre staff in my field notes: "A few things recently made me wonder about the training and capacity of the (junior) nurses here. I had to re-bandage a child's leg that was badly burned and attracting flies. It was from a cooking fire (charcoal fires are low, and kids sometimes trip and fall on them). It's a pretty common type of injury/accident here, but you might think a nurse would be able to prevent it, or at least be taking better measures for it to heal without infection. After I brought over the bandage, N. ([a different child] J.'s mum) asked me about whether we had medicine, because J. had a crack on his foot that seemed infected. Again, it just made me wonder about her nursing knowledge as well as access to supplies and care." While there is some judgment in this field note (prevention!), these kind of observations helped me to understand that for junior unaccredited staff, the difference in status and access between themselves and their patients was not very great.

### Informal Health Care Providers

*Traditional Birth Attendants (TBAs)*

The WHO defines a TBA as "a person who assists the mother during childbirth, and who initially acquired her skills by delivering babies herself or through an apprenticeship to other TBAs" (WHO, 1992, p. 4). This definition is consistent with the women who practised as TBAs in Amuru. I learned about their roles and practice from childbearing women and from other health providers and administrators, as well as from 10 TBAs themselves during focus groups (also discussed in Rudrum 2016b). The TBAs, all women in their 50s and 60s, told me they had learned through *experience*, by *necessity*, and by *taking courage*. In previous generations, they explained, all older women would have been expected to be able to assist at a birth. In the context of low life expectancy, these women were all elders in their communities.

I started each TBA focus group by asking how the women had first learned birth skills, and each shared a detailed story. To explain the process of becoming a TBA, Dorota simply explained, "Me, I first saw it from big people [elders] and felt it is all courage. And then I felt that I should also have that courage and help pregnant women." Amaya told the story of the first birth at which she had assisted, which was before she had given birth to any child of her own, suggesting she was still a girl:

> One time I found a woman knelt down, next to a house, so I went and knelt near her, and when the child came, I waited and received the baby. There were two babies. I waited and received the second one too, and also then I removed the placenta. I went to the big people [elders] and said that the woman who knelt there had delivered twins. So that courage, I have had it forever now.

The TBAs I spoke with had all participated in organized training (funded by NGOs and often delivered via health centres) at various points over the past three decades. However, in each case, often by telling a story, they identified local and informal experience as the way they had become TBAs.

While the term *TBAs* is often deployed in contrast to SBAs, defined as those with formal training, this can be misleading. The contrast is deceptive because TBAs certainly have birth skills, often including skills useful in a difficult labour such as a breech or multiple birth. As well, not all of those providing care in health centres fit the official definition of SBAs. As I described earlier, those who worked as nurse aides were, like TBAs, laypeople. They had been hired from within the community without formal qualifications and were trained on the job to perform health care, including delivery care. This is often overlooked in the dichotomy between "traditional" and "skilled" birth attendants. When it came to traditional practices not rooted in Western medicine, the TBAs I spoke with mentioned these with both positive and negative assessments. For example, the practice of using charred grass (*raah*) to cut the umbilical cord was regarded as still useful in the absence of a clean and sharp razorblade. In contrast, one participant mentioned a past response to a baby who was not breathing might be a gentle hit on the head with the flat part of a hoe in tandem with inviting men to smoke in proximity; the practice of holding the infant upside down and patting its back was seen, perhaps not surprisingly, as a better solution. I was, however, somewhat surprised to hear dismissive laughter around the past use of various traditional herbs.

The childbearing women who I spoke with primarily looked to TBAs for labour support, rather than for a broader role of support and care throughout pregnancy. They mainly discussed the labour support that they sought from TBAs as a backup to or substitute for clinical support in a health facility. Jacky told me about how a lack of transportation and cell phone network access made going to the health centre impossible. In contrast, Pauline, who had one baby and had lost her older child at about five to malaria, delivered in the health centre but told me: "If it [labour] had been abrupt, I would have delivered at home with the help of a TBA." Margaret reflected on her TBA-assisted home birth saying, "It was distance and the problem of transport. Otherwise, I would have delivered at the hospital [health centre] like my fellow women." Her view that health centre birth was a norm among her peers at this time was prevalent. In fact, of 45 participants in this stage (35 interviews and 10 focus group participants), 10 had given birth outside a health centre or hospital.

TBAs play an important yet contentious role in maternity care in Uganda. Many births outside a health facility are attended by a TBA, yet TBAs have a precarious status. Because of shifts in approaches and informal policy pronouncements, identifying the Ugandan policy approach to TBAs is challenging. While major Ugandan newspapers *The Monitor* and *The New Vision*, as well as the British paper *The Guardian*, reported a 2009 ban on TBAs,[3] I could not identify policy documents to indicate that such a ban had ever taken place. During my time at the health centre, I learned that the situation governing TBAs was, in fact, unclear. There had never been an official written policy banning TBAs, but there had been a number of speeches or documents referring to such a ban.

---

3 See, for example, *The Guardian*'s articles "Traditional Birth Attendants Show No Sign of Abandoning Their Work in Katine" (Malinga, 2010) and "Should Uganda Ban Traditional Birth Attendants?" (Murigi & Ford, 2010); *The New Vision*, the state-run newspaper, "Revisiting the Policy on Traditional Birth Attendants" (Kabayambi, 2013); or *The Monitor*, a leading independent newspaper, "Why Traditional Birth Attendants Will Keep Thriving" (Tegulle, 2013).

It was reported that the UMOH was resolved to ban TBAs by 2015 as an HIV-reduction strategy (Mafaranga, 2013); no such ban has happened. The government's strong anti-TBA stance, coupled with lack of any concrete guidelines, challenged administrators working in communities where TBAs practise.

Writing before the time of the presidential statement against TBAs, Kyomugisha (2008) summarized, "Caught between tolerating the need for their service and seeing it as illegal, the government occasionally openly discourages it" (p. 21). The UMOH, for example, had circulated an edict to NGOs asking them to stop training TBAs (Murigi & Ford, 2010). In our interview, the clinical officer in-charge at the health centre, Jonas, explained the situation as follows:

> Actually, what transpired in the past that they, the TBAs, should not conduct deliveries, it was not a policy; it was not a law, neither was it a bylaw, but it was a statement, just, from the president that came out after [a] woman died in labour in eastern Uganda. So the president said "this was done, she died in the hand of a TBA, so with immediately effect, all TBAs must not conduct deliveries." So this was just a statement, there was no documentation. That was why it became very difficult to implement such a statement, to start working.

Here, Jonas clarifies that there was no policy per se but that a statement from the president following this maternal death was nevertheless influential on future decision making. The lack of a clear policy governing the role of TBAs in health care provision made it difficult, and at times confusing, for local health care administrators and indeed TBAs themselves to know how to proceed. Health care administrators worked with TBAs, acknowledging that they would continue to play a role. This is in part because the capacity for SBAs at every birth does not exist: "It has been argued that the generally poor functionality of the health system means that TBAs will continue to remain a source of care for many especially in rural areas of Uganda" (Turinawe et al., 2016, p. 2–3). The health care centre officially encouraged TBAs to refer all patients, refraining from providing delivery services, while acknowledging that this was more idealistic than descriptive. The TBAs I spoke with simultaneously accepted referral as a positive role and acknowledged it as not always possible. Joanna spoke of referral when telling us about a teacher's wife who did not want to go to the health centre for delivery. She told Joanna that she feared the child would be Odoch, that is, born foot first, because she had been told this during ANC at the health centre. Joanna said she examined her and reassured her that the baby's position was normal. When she went into labour, the woman was frightened and asked Joanna to stay at home with her, but Joanna refused and escorted her to the health centre, along with the woman's mother. The baby was born without complication. Joanna offered this as an illustration of the larger point that it is now no longer acceptable to deliver at home if it is not necessary and to describe how she complied with the advice to play a referral role.

However, in light of the continued need for their services, TBAs with whom I spoke suggested they needed some support for safety at deliveries. They identified the following supplies as necessary: rubber boots (for the rainy season and for protection from snakes when walking at night), gloves (for hygiene), and flashlights (for travel and as a light source during delivery care). In addition, TBAs told me that they wanted to be trained how to ascertain a woman's HIV status from the ANC card (since they couldn't read). This is an example of how illiteracy influenced the role of texts in coordinating care translocally: the intention of recording HIV test results on a card that women carried was to allow care providers at a later date and in a different location to check these results. However, the ANC card text could not coordinate knowledge of women's HIV status in this way for TBAs, since they could not read and had not been trained to identify the results. The many barriers to accessing formal delivery care discussed throughout this book contribute to the ongoing need for the birth work provided by TBAs despite the confused and negative policy environment and the lack of support for their work.

### The Village Health Team (VHT)

The VHT members were another group of laypeople who did health work with pregnant women. The VHT program is a UMOH initiative introduced in 2001 using unpaid volunteer community health workers. Members of the VHT, who receive some training, are considered to be an HCI, the lowest level of health centre. That is, while they do not work out of a physical health facility, they are the first point of contact between individuals and the health care system (UMOH, 2010, p. 9). Their role is to provide a bridge to formal health care. They are also health educators and mobilizers, informing their community of upcoming outreach visits and ensuring that people are present on such days.

In describing the VHT's role, the UMOH draws on a discourse of responsibilization (Foley, 2008; Rossiter, 2012; Ruhl, 1999). This discourse leverages statistics on disease prevention to place responsibility for poor health or disease outbreaks on individual or community behaviours. For example, a training document claims that "in Uganda, over

75% of the diseases are preventable if only people changed and adopted appropriate and well known behaviors geared towards better health" (UMOH, 2010, p. 7). This practice shifts responsibility for poor health outcomes away from the inadequate and poorly funded health system, and towards individuals and communities. The rationale for the VHT makes claims about empowerment and taking responsibility: "Community participation and empowerment is a strategy that enables communities to take responsibility for their own health and wellbeing and to participate actively in the management of their local health services" (UMOH, 2010, p. 7). This focus shifts the blame for health problems to individuals and communities, rather than health systems or other public sectors. The VHT program is intended to be a means of facilitating access to health care while at the same time reducing demands on the formal health care system by improving health within communities. Participants primarily mentioned the VHT in relation to registration for the mama kits (discussed in detail in chapter 4) but also as a source of information.

### Transportation, Nutrition, and Work

Among the aspects of everyday life shaping pregnancy and maternity care, finding transportation, managing nutrition, and balancing the need for rest with agricultural work (and the need for an income) were the three most prominent aspects, in terms of both the frequency with which they were mentioned and their potential impact on health and health care. These factors of course are interrelated, with access to money facilitating access to better nutrition and transportation, and the exhortation to rest adequately made difficult by the need for food and money.

### *Transportation*

Transportation connected the communities where pregnant women lived to the health centres where antenatal and birthing care were provided, and therefore facilitated access to maternity health care. However, transportation challenges were complex and, at times, insurmountable. The challenge of transportation affects the location of birth and thereby the type of attendant present and is widely understood as logistically and financially difficult to the extent that it affects birth practices and outcomes in Uganda (Kyomuhendo, 2003; Knudsen, 2003; Parkhurst et al., 2006). Transportation was not one problem but was multidimensional. It impeded an increase in health centre delivery, as ongoing reliance on TBAs at the time of birth was connected to the difficulty of transportation, particularly for those living in remote communities or delivering at night.

A central road linked Amuru, where Lacor HCIII was located, to Otwee, the district headquarters, and other trading centres. To the southeast, this road connected to the Juba road, a major north-south route on which Lacor Hospital is located. The roads themselves were narrow, poorly surfaced, and unmaintained. During the rainy season, they could quickly become impassable: in a field note near the start of the rainy season, written after an attempt to return home, I wrote, "Once the array of stopped semis jackknifed across the narrow road made it evident that we would not be able to pass, we turned around, and spent the evening in Gulu, where we got a room at the Acholi Inn, went for Ethiopian food, and contemplated whether we would be holed up in Amuru for the next five months." Private car or truck ownership was rare: short distances were covered by foot, bicycle, or *boda*, longer trips could be taken by shared van-taxi or *boda*, and emergency transportation was via ambulances.

Ambulances, typically converted Toyota Land Cruisers, were used to transport patients who needed medical assistance beyond the health centre's scope, taking them to hospital. Unlike ambulances in wealthier settings, these are summoned not by patients but by staff at the lower-level health care facility. They provide transportation only – they are staffed by a driver and are not equipped with medical equipment or with supplies, outside of medical masks, which were passed out to me and to patients when one of the patients being transported had presumed measles during an outbreak in 2019. At government-run facilities, however, lack of a vehicle or money for fuel hindered emergency transport. Lacor HCIII had no vehicle, but depended on ambulance service via Lacor Hospital, which, in my observation and as communicated to me by Jonas and Peter, the DHO, was reliable (particularly in contrast with the lack of service at government-run facilities). Management had been able to improve emergency transportation in response to an incident in which a nighttime ambulance delay led to a "near-miss" for a labouring woman; both she and her baby survived, but she had to have a hysterectomy. After that, an improvement was made to the procedure for contacting night ambulance drivers such that night drivers were required to be present at Lacor Hospital during their on-call shifts to ensure their ability to respond to calls from the rural health centres (Jonas, personal communication, 2012). This system nevertheless meant a delay as the ambulance had to be dispatched from Lacor Hospital near Gulu, rather than being available on site.

For personal transportation to health care, *boda-bodas* played a large role. A *boda-boda* (motorcycle taxi) was not an ideal mode of transportation for a labouring woman, and advanced labour could sometimes make it impossible. The more pervasive challenge, however, was not being able to get a *boda*. People often contacted drivers by walking to an intersection where drivers were known to wait; women might also gather in advance the phone numbers of drivers they knew. Since costs rose in relation to distance travelled, remote women were more greatly affected. The difficulty of contacting drivers after dark and their reluctance to travel at night reduced transportation accessibility for labouring women. Poor road conditions made travel at night unsafe; drivers also reportedly feared "bad people" and felt more susceptible to crime if travelling at night. Weather also affected transportation because during heavy rain, travel was difficult, uncomfortable, and hard to arrange.

One participant, Elizabeth, when asked which people were most important to a pregnant woman, said the *boda-boda* driver. When my RA laughed, she conceded that perhaps her husband was most important. However, her initial mention of a *boda* driver was revealing. Without a *boda-boda* driver, a woman might not be able to deliver at the health centre. She would labour at home, supported by whoever was available.

The remote location of many households contributed to transportation difficulties. As farmers, people in Amuru often situated their homes in proximity to their land, rather than with a view to accessing roads or trading centres. The narrow paths that households were located on were not accessible by car or truck, and even motorcycle access could be difficult when paths were overgrown or wet. While the distance to the road was regarded as walkable, walking any distance can be difficult when heavily pregnant or in labour, and, once a woman reached the road, transportation was not always available, for reasons described above. Even in the nearest villages, people talked about transportation to the health centre as an issue, but distance contributed to whether women would attend ANC or deliver in a health centre. If transportation to the local health centre was often a challenge, transportation to a full-service hospital was generally an insurmountable one. The trip was too long and too costly for most people to manage independently.

The connection between transportation challenges and birthing at home was articulated by Jacky, who lived in the remote village Teddi. She told me her birth story as follows:

> I started to feel labour pain in the evening when the sun was down, and it was hard to get a *boda* [motorcycle taxi]. So one has to call a *boda* from

Amuru to take you to the hospital, but also the phone network here is very poor, so they had to look for the network – one has to go and stand on an anthill [to get any cell phone reception]. So, by the time they called the *boda* to reach here, I had already delivered because the labour started so urgently. I had to deliver with the help of the trained TBA who was around here.

Her story, like many I heard, made it difficult to tease out truly precipitous labour as a factor separate from numerous delays. For Jacky, relying on a TBA for labour support was circumstantial, rather than part of a birth plan, preference, or deliberate choice.

Some women travelled to ANC appointments by bicycle, either doubled by their partner or riding the bike themselves. Women were advised not to ride a bike themselves when their pregnancies were advanced. It was not typical for every household to have a bike; couples sometimes borrowed from a sibling or neighbour. Bike ownership was gendered such that when a household owned a bike, it generally belonged to a man. Overall, women were less geographically mobile and had less access to transportation than men did.

The practice of living on site at the health centre reduced the transportation challenge for health workers themselves, in many instances. Health workers did, despite better access than most, experience and sympathize with transportation challenges. I knew the DHO, Peter, from being introduced to him on his visits to the health centre and from running into him at various health-related workshops and conferences in Gulu town, where he lived, commuting to work at his offices near a rural government-run health centre. By the time of our formal interview, however, we'd had to cancel at least twice: once because the rain was too heavy for me to travel via *boda*, and once because he was not able to use his car for some reason. When I asked him about transportation as a dimension of access to care, he acknowledged, "It's a challenge everywhere. You have seen the roads. You have seen the inability to have means of transport." He went on to ask, "If it is a challenge to us, what would be the magnitude of the challenge at the community level?" A government employee, he felt that the necessary resources were unlikely to come via government funding and that the best solution might be a collective one in which communities contributed to the cost of fuel and maintenance. He acknowledged, however, that such as solution would also face many challenges, including competing expenses.

Increasing the number of operational health centres would mitigate the transportation problem, as it would many of the care challenges I encountered. If each health centre in Amuru that was designated as an HCII or HCIII was operational to their prescribed levels, most women could walk to ANC, saving them the work, expense, and risk of arranging transport. I invited participants to discuss recommendations, and they suggested various approaches to improving transportation to health care, including pooling savings to purchase fuel for ambulances (for the government hospital), organizing emergency community funds for women without the means to pay for a *boda*, and providing a shuttle service from health centres that could not provide appropriate care to a health centre with adequate maternity care services. Transportation problems in Amuru sub-county were multifaceted and, as such, require interventions that factor in these multiple elements. Interventions that isolate one transportation barrier are limited in their ability to effect change. For example, programs that distribute *boda-boda* vouchers (described in Pariyo et al., 2011) address cost but not other transportation barriers. The major roads in the north have improved markedly since the study period; however, the challenges of serving a large sub-county with inadequate services remained. A 2019 article reported an ambulance to person ratio of 1:33,600 in the Acholi sub-region (focusing on government-provided services) with no government ambulance in all of Amuru district (Owich, 2019).

### LACK OF CAPACITY TO PROVIDE CARE AT SUB-COUNTY HEALTH CENTRES

Otwee HCIII, a government-run facility in the district, was an example of a health centre that was not functioning to its designated capacity. Because of its problems with service delivery, participants who lived near there would bypass it in order to reach more reliable care at Lacor HCIII. None of the 45 participants reported having given birth to their most recent child there. The DHO, Peter, lived at least 50 kilometres away in the neighbouring district, Gulu, but had his office near Otwee Health Centre and was responsible for its administration. He described an encounter he had had with a group of local women who, frustrated over the (total) absence of beds in the maternity ward, had formed a group to barricade the road out of the district headquarters, demanding to speak to him before he left for his home in Gulu that day. They made their case for beds in the maternity ward; however, Peter reportedly explained that he had prioritized trained staff over beds, being unable to provide both. He asked them, rhetorically, whether if they stayed at home there would be a bed (there would not) and emphasized that skilled staff members were the most important intervention the health centre could make in delivery care. When patients opt to travel to a farther health centre, it is known as bypassing; although the term suggests choice and agency, when the health system is weak, the closer health centre is often not a viable option.

In May 2013, five health workers at Otwee Health Centre, a government-run health facility, were charged with "neglect of duty and absenteeism from work place without permission at expense of tax payers' life" (Gilbert & Otika, 2013, para 6; Women of Uganda Network, 2013). Absenteeism is sometimes attributed to delayed or erratic pay (Ackers et al., 2016). A volunteer working with a social accountability group had been the one to raise the alarm on their absenteeism, working through authorities to contact the police. Inoperational health centres caused distress and additional work for pregnant women and others needing care. One practice of IE research is to "investigate that which informants experience as problematic, troubling, and contradictory" (Bisaillon, 2012, p. 609). The instances of activism described here bolster the evidence in interviews and focus groups indicating that lack of capacity to provide health care to specified levels was a priority issue for participants and other people in Amuru. The clear demands of local activists indicate that patients saw themselves as able to shape how formal care was organized and not as passive recipients of whatever care was provided. These activist demands support my finding that when women stayed home to deliver, it wasn't always because of a preference for home and the care available there; it was sometimes an indictment of, or a result of the challenge of accessing, the health care environment.

*Nutrition and Work*

Participants often paired nutrition and work as aspects of self-care during pregnancy. Eating well and avoiding heavy or prolonged physical labour were known to be important to taking care of the health of mother and unborn baby; this was emphasized in health talks and during ANC, yet in some instances participants found this difficult. The focus on avoiding heavy work and seeking nutrition indicated that the local livelihood, subsistence farming, was significant in shaping approaches to care at birth. All capable family members farmed by hand with a heavy hoe, and as farming was the principle livelihood, avoiding this work was challenging. Poverty also contributed to the difficulty of adequate rest and nutrition. Participants reported that pregnant women would sometimes work for their neighbours, typically at farm work, to save for good food and for basic supplies necessary at the time of birth; the need to provide these supplies contributed to the difficulty of avoiding heavy work or getting adequate rest during pregnancy.

Participants paired seeking good nutrition and avoiding work because both were well-known pieces of self-care advice and because the one depended on the other. Eating well depended on having a good yield, varied crops, and some money for store-bought food such as dried fish, oil, sugar, salt, and perhaps eggs or meat. For most, good nutrition depended on hard work, an irony of the self-care advice that was pointed out by various participants.

Rest and nutrition are important to pregnant women across social contexts. I nevertheless found it frustrating to see such basic needs dominating women's and health care worker's efforts and couldn't help but reflect on how such a focus is inevitably at the expense of something else. I observed that knowledge of the advice to avoid arduous work and seek good nutrition overshadowed other relevant knowledge, such as how to recognize pregnancy danger signs that indicate a need to seek care. When asked about caring for pregnancy, no other risk factors were mentioned by mothers. While workshops on nutrition were hosted at the health centre, workshops on other aspects of healthy pregnancy were not held, to my knowledge. Similarly, at times, the need for women to prioritize their work at home and on the land left little room for the work of care seeking, a problem that women returned to often in discussing the work of pregnancy.

While some could delegate work to supportive others – husbands, older children, or co-wives – others were frustrated by the lack of help. Leah said that some men made resting or eating well more difficult for their partners:

> Men are different. Some think women pretend when you tell him you are not able [to work] so he will ask you to dig equally, because the child is in the womb and not in your hand [laughter].

Such expectations contributed to the difficulty of avoiding overwork in pregnancy. Janice also mentioned overwork. When I met her, I noted she looked tired and older than 24. In the interview, she recounted that during delivery she repeatedly passed out with exhaustion. Even now, six months after the birth of her third child, she said, she was exhausted.

Preparations for delivery and planning for care were forms of work in themselves, in addition to agricultural or other subsistence/income-generating work. Some participants turned to income-generating work to be able to buy required supplies for delivery. As well as heavy work such as digging someone's field, this could be, for those with the capital and resources to arrange it, lighter work such as cooking and selling snacks. Participants identified the necessary supplies for delivering at the health centre and receiving the baby as including a plastic bed cover on which to labour (to contribute to a sterile environment), clothes and cloths for the baby, lamp paraffin for night waking, and prepared food items (such as food that needed to be ground). Women also mudded (or "smeared") the floor of their huts in preparation for the new arrival, applying a paste of dung and water to make a clean and smooth surface. This was explained as important because the new baby was like a guest or because guests could be expected after the baby's arrival. In any case, mudding the floor was home maintenance that had to be done periodically, and there would be no time for it with a newborn. Women prepared *simsim* [sesame] for making pasted foods and millet for porridge; again, grinding these was labour intensive and would be difficult with a new baby. Participants told me about all of this in answer to a question about what they needed to do to prepare for delivery; they mostly considered obtaining supplies and preparing foods or the home to be part of the work of pregnancy. Of course, it was more difficult for some participants than for others. The difficulty of avoiding arduous work was linked to the need to purchase and prepare supplies for the pregnancy, birth, and baby's arrival.

The region has a dry and a rainy season; while the rainy season adds to transportation costs and logistics, the dry season exacerbates the challenge of healthy eating; these dynamics also occur in southern Uganda (MacVicar et al., 2017). The "lean months" that some participants described contributed to the difficulty of avoiding work and ensuring nutrition. When the last harvest had been eaten or sold and the new crop was not yet ready, nutrition became a challenge. Maureen, who was struggling financially, listed tomatoes, eggs, and milk as foods that would contribute to good nutrition during pregnancy but that were difficult to obtain. In a difficult interview, she spoke about seeing well-fed children with a sense of envy, telling me, "In this month, hunger is much." In a focus group discussion, Betty said, on the topic of food, that "nutrition is good, as they tell us … But it is not easy … While the children are hungry, eggs cannot be eaten [by mothers]. It is impossible." For these women, eating nutritious foods during pregnancy competed with providing adequate food to their children. Like any mother, they prioritized the well-being of their children.

The challenge of nutrition was linked to the post-conflict setting in that the production of some foods took longer, or was more expensive, to re-establish. This was the case with livestock, tree fruit, and avocados, for example. During the war, people would grow crops that were difficult to raid or would sell their produce quickly to an urban intermediary. Finnström (2008) writes, "Eventually, the short-term coping strategy of selling off harvests and then buying food will make people increasingly entangled with the wider market economy and its fluctuations, or even dependent on relief distribution" (p. 36). Participants also described to me this continued pattern of selling off much of a crop early. Although it was no longer a strategy to avoid raids, selling the bulk of a crop at the time of harvest impacted access to nutritious foods. Participants also looked for humanitarian-aid food support such as they had experienced in the camps. For example, Hazel recalled a nutritionally enhanced flour that included soy that was distributed around 2004, when people were returning home from IDP camps. She said, "It gives expectant mothers and the baby strength, and nowadays they don't give." When food given as aid is successfully framed as superior in some way to locally available foods, its withdrawal can cause worry. Others recommended that the government or health centre should provide sugar or other food supports. For instance, Nightie, a focus group participant in Lujoro said that "actually when it comes to delivery, there are so many problems, because we don't have the capacity to take care of ourselves. When we deliver, sometimes we even don't have what to eat, so the hospital should try to support a little." McElroy (2012) found that while reliance on food aid was not desirable, the vulnerability of children (her study's focus) to nutritional deprivation was such that targeted intervention for pregnant and breastfeeding women and young children should be considered (p. 147). The context of previous humanitarian aid in the area, particularly in IDP camps and during their disbandment, shaped childbearing women's expectations and recommendations with regard to food support.

Ensuring good nutrition and avoiding heavy work were also emphasized in my discussions with formal health care providers. While they promoted the view that maintaining good nutrition and avoiding heavy work were important, health administrators and workers (Peter, Jonas, Amy, Grace, Gloria, and Dorothy) felt food insecurity or lack of nutritious food was something women could manage, even in the poorest family, an optimism that contrasted with the perspectives of childbearing women. They argued that every family would have some land to plant, noting that Amuru is a fertile and productive area. They told me that they talked to women about using food storage services and growing a kitchen garden in their compound. They shared a perspective that families could manage their resources better to avoid shortfalls. In contrast, many women emphasized that having good food to eat during pregnancy and birth was very challenging. Health care providers seemed to be sharing a message of responsibilization when it came to nutrition and did not believe that poverty was so extreme that good nutrition would be difficult.

As well as being a factor in healthy pregnancy, the need to work and provide good nutrition could also lead to delays in seeking care. One participant, Hope, laughed when telling her birth story, in which a series of pressing household tasks led to a delay in arranging transportation to the health centre. Hope lived near the health centre and had the money to pay for the short *boda-boda* ride. However, when she went into labour at a friend's home, she worried about leaving home without having prepared firewood for her children so that they could cook. Hope was prepared to both educate and entertain with her birth story:

> Then I ran, with my boy, after he had put some beans on the fire, then I said, "you follow me." I came home, and split firewood very fast. After I split firewood, the baby's head seemed to be down already, and [laughs] pain increased and it was much … I said, I will first get some potatoes. It [the pain] had subsided, so I poured water into a basin. I had bathed during the day but I said, "I will bathe only here" [indicates washing between her legs, laughs]. I had everything packed, ready [i.e., her supplies for the birth at the health centre]. I started getting potatoes from the garden, very fast, then I went to cut [harvest] *simsim* [sesame] I had sowed here. I cut five handfuls, and when I had cut the *simsim* my labour increased so much it was impossible. I sent the children that "you go and call this woman[4] to come, I am going to the hospital [health centre]." The lady ran and came. I had bathed, I said, "I will put my clothes on," then my waters burst (*pii oo*). They ran to call a motorcycle. The baby then came out! [laughs].

Delivering at the health centre was Hope's plan, but she had other priorities. As with many other participants, going to the health centre would mean leaving behind older children, and she needed to ensure they would be able to cope. Of her older children, three had been born at home and another two at the health centre, so she was comfortable with both home and facility birth. Since that birth, she had suffered two miscarriages; when I closed our interview by asking what else she would like me to know, she said that child health after six months needed to be considered, as between leaving school at noon and dinner time, children often had nothing to eat. Later on the day of our interview, I ran into Hope, harvesting *simsim*. Her story helped to situate birth for me within the daily rhythm of women's lives, much of which involved the work of food procurement.

Pregnancy is a time of vulnerability for women, as the changes in the body introduce new health risks and women and families adapt to economic and time pressures. The struggles to maintain basic nutrition and rest during pregnancy and the difficulty of obtaining necessary services

---

4 The woman was a neighbour who Hope said was not a TBA but "works almost like a TBA."

and goods, such as transportation and birth supplies, rendered women in Amuru particularly vulnerable in the time during and around pregnancy. Such forces can be considered acts of structural violence, violent because of the harms they cause and structural because they are embedded in social and economic institutions. Finnström argues that physical violence occurs "when access to transportation is very unevenly distributed, keeping large segments of a populations at the same place with mobility a monopoly of the select few" (Galtung, 1969, p. 169, as cited in Finnström, 2008, p. 145). As pertains to transportation for health care in Amuru, poverty, neglected rural and northern infrastructure, and poor health care infrastructure conspired to make access to transportation an issue that brought violence and impaired the capacity of women to meet their basic human needs. These everyday issues of transport, food, and work had significant impacts on the health of childbearing women in Amuru sub-county. While the challenges of transportation, nutrition, and work were part of ordinary life in post-conflict Amuru, such challenges were structurally constituted and were therefore modifiable.

# Chapter Four

# Charity and Control: When Help Requires Compliance

## Introduction

In the first of my interviews with mothers in northern Uganda, partici-pants talked about receiving or not receiving a mama kit from the health centre. It turned out that this small gift to mothers played a large role in linking local and extra-local concerns and practices in relation to mater-nity care. In this chapter, I examine differing accounts of the purpose of the mama kits, with attention to their uneven distribution. I describe the work that pregnant women, VHT members, and formal health staff conducted in relation to the kits' registration and distribution. The com-peting needs of NGOs, the health centre, and birthing women shaped access to resources and care. Ideologies of scarcity, responsibility, and deservedness characterized the relationship between the mama kits and maternity care.

The mama kits were a bag of basic baby supplies given to women after delivery. The kits contained a bar of soap, a washing basin, towels, diaper cream, and eye ointment. They were supplied as a project of the Japa-nese Red Cross and the Uganda Red Cross. Pregnant women were to register and receive a card (different from the ANC card) to receive the kit; registration was by VHT members appointment by the Red Cross.

The work of Marcel Mauss is foundational to sociological and anthro-pological theories of gift giving and to understanding the meaning of gifts in different social contexts. Mauss (1925, 1990) discusses the requirement for reciprocity and contests a framing of gifts as freely given: "In theory such gifts are voluntary but in fact they are given and repaid under obligation" (p. 3). Gifts to the poor share features of other gift giving but introduce an element of justice: "Alms are the result on the one hand of a moral idea about gifts and wealth and on the other of an idea about sacrifice" (Mauss, 1925, 1990, p. 15). His work was taken up by Claude Levi-Strauss (1965), who viewed gifts as inherently political in nature, playing a non-material role as instruments for "influence, power, sympathy, status, emotion" (p. 65). Levi-Strauss (1965) argued that "the skillful game of exchange consists of a complex totality of manoeuver, conscious or unconscious, in order to gain security and to fortify one's self against risks incurred through alliances and rivalry" (p. 65). Sociological analysis of gift giving has also been taken up in contemporary development studies, such as by Stirrat and Henkel (1997) who make the case that in development as elsewhere, there is no such thing as a free gift (see also Mawdsley, 2012). Rather than representing a one-way flow of goods and altruism, charitable gifts in fact bind the global north and global south in complex and problematic ways. In the field of maternal health, gift giving has primarily been theorized in relation to surrogacy and its potential for altruism or commodification (Ragoné, 1999), along somewhat similar lines to discussions of other potential "gifts of life" such as organs or blood (Titmuss, 1970). Gifts that are given to newly parturient women in health care settings are also socially significant. There are other health systems in which mothers can bring home a gift of baby care items; the meaning and impact of such gifts varies depending on the social and political context in which they are offered, as I have explored in a co-authored article in *The Sociology of Health and Illness* (Rudrum et al., 2016).

In tracing practices surrounding the mama kits, it became clear to me that they functioned as a linkage between local and extra-local relations, involving many disparate actors in maternity care and birth, including individual childbearing women; VHT members; staff at the health centre, itself run by an international NGO; government health administrators; and international and national NGOs. Significantly, TBAs were not involved in the registration for or distribution of the mama kits. Indeed, for childbearing women, TBAs' lack of access to this resource distinguished their care at delivery from that offered by SBAs at health centres. The discursive and material impact of the mama kits was a feature of how maternity care was organized, controlled, and negotiated in Amuru.

IE focuses on identifying how contemporary ruling relations are constituted through "the complex of extra-local relations that provide in contemporary societies a specialization of organization, control, and initiative" (Smith, 1990, p. 6). These forms of organization and control include "bureaucracy, administration, management, professional organization, and the media" (Smith, 2002, p. 6). This form of social organization is "objectified" in that it is external to and "independent of particular individuals and particularized relations" (Smith, 2005, p. 14). While a rural sub-Saharan setting such as Amuru means fewer encounters with bureaucracy, mass media, or other forms of translocal organization than in the global north, such forms are nevertheless present and influential. This was evident in features of bureaucracy exemplified by the mama kit registration card and the ANC card, as well as in forms of professional organization within and between the VHT, health centres, and NGOs. As I examine the role of the mama kits project in the coordination of maternity care and childbirth, I pay particular attention to such forms of organization and control.

## A Reward for Care or a Gift to the Vulnerable? Divergent Ideas on the Mama Kit's Role

For the women I spoke with, the mama kits were important and valued. They functioned as a form of access to items necessary for post-partum recovery and newborn care. It was this necessity, in the context of poverty and limited access to resources, that allowed the kits to be leveraged into an influential role.

In contrast to their agreement regarding the utility and importance of the mama kits, ideas on the purpose of the mama kits project varied strikingly, as did women's experiences of registration issues and receiving or not receiving a mama kit. Some said that the mama kits were distributed as an incentive or reward for attending a full program of ANC, described as three or four visits; others said it was as an incentive or reward for delivering at a health facility or saw it as support, whether for new mothers generally or for particular groups of mothers. While all women were aware of and wanted to receive the mama kits, at least 20 of 45 women interviewed did not receive a kit or received only part of the kit's contents. As I work to make sense of these divergent accounts and experiences, I examine the texts and talk of participants' descriptions of the mama kits' purpose and the work involved in registering for and receiving them. In particular, I describe how, because they were often perceived to be a reward or incentive for attending ANC or delivering in a health centre, these resources shaped the ways in which maternity care was sought and accessed.

### The Mama Kit as Creating and Rewarding Compliance with ANC

Among participants, attending ANC – and having the ANC card to demonstrate that they had done so – was seen as a "key" to health centre delivery. Without this key, one might be turned away or "chased," as women described it. In describing receiving the mama kit as dependent on attending ANC, women emphasized the importance of health workers' message to attend ANC. Betty, who had not received a kit and who mentioned problems with registration, saw the use of the mama kit as simultaneously coercive and helpful. She told me, "It is true that when you don't go for ANC three times, they don't give you [the mama kit]. They are right, because we women need orders." Betty understood the gift as a mode of "giving orders" and accepted this practice. Attaching provision of the mama kit to women's participation in ANC was a way for the health centre to exert power over women's ANC attendance. Provision of the kits as a reward for compliance with care reinforced power differences between care providers and birthing women.

A first-time mother living near the health centre, Rose, explained that staff had told her she received the mama kit because she attended ANC:

> They said we followed measurements [ANC] very well. Some people don't follow measurements in the hospital [health centre] well, they don't finish, but for us we finished ours, and we saw our health [tested for HIV and learned status].

The language in this quotation, on measurements and on hospital, may require some explanation. Acero, the RA, explained that attending ANC was referred to as *pime*, which means measurement but was also used to mean a check-up. During ANC, fundal height was measured to monitor the fetus's development and to estimate due dates. Participants typically referred to both a health centre and a hospital in the same way, as an *ot yat*; however, it was very clear when they were talking about the hospital, since going to a full-service hospital such as Lacor Hospital in Gulu was somewhat exceptional, as it required leaving the district at considerable expense. As Rose emphasized, compliance was rewarded with a mama kit, as well as with praise from care providers. Earlier, I introduced the idea that providing or withholding health care, and the way care is offered, can signal messages about citizenship (Sinding, 2010). The mama kits were one mechanism signalling that that there were good and bad ways of participating in care, and a woman's approach would be rewarded by inclusion or exclusion. Being a good citizen through seeking health care relates to responsibilization discourses: "the mundane striving for 'good' or 'perfect' health involves intensive 'work on the self' or self-governance, and despite the language of empowerment and freedom, this striving for health entails compulsion, added responsibilities to others, and often punishment and social exclusion in the case of those who fail to conform" (Petersen et al., 2010, p. 392). A participant, Rose, emphasized that HIV testing (examined in detail in chapter 5) was an important reason why ANC was encouraged by health workers and other public health means.

Elizabeth, another participant living near the health centre, told me that ANC was promoted for women regardless of where they would eventually give birth. Her newborn had been born at the health centre and had struggled to breathe at the time of birth; she believed he would not have survived without the assistance provided at the health centre. She had received a mama kit after giving birth. Elizabeth explained:

> You should have gone for ANC four times in order for you to get those things. When you have not yet delivered, even those who are not going to give birth from the health centre, it is good if you follow what they have told you to do and finish the ANC very well.

Here, Elizabeth identifies the mama kits project as reinforcing the importance of attending ANC, regardless of where a woman plans to deliver.

The mama kit project sets apart its recipients as different from the general population, who are constructed as not in need, as well as from their benefactors, who have the capacity to give. Women are targeted both for their poverty and for what is oftentimes construed as their reluctance to seek formal care. The attempt to improve the numbers of women receiving formal care is a form of intervention that occurs in the context of high maternal mortality.

Relying on material incentives to improve rates of seeking health care is linked to ideas of compliance. The constructs of compliance and adherence, both referring to "how well patients follow health advice" (Mykhalovskiy et al., 2004, p. 316) have been critiqued by sociologists since the 1970s as forms of medical control that rely on notions of the patient as a passive subject (Trostle, 1988; Zola, 1981). In revisiting the concept, Mykhalovskiy et al. (2004) note that in contemporary health practices, power cannot be conceived solely as top-down and held by physicians. In global health, the critique of adherence is resonant for the impacts of a "moral calculus" in which the documented or presumed non-adherence of a population group is used as a form of blame for drug-resistance or as an excuse to not extend costly and complex medical treatments, such as for HIV (Crane, 2013). Compliance discourse also tends to have different dimensions in global health contexts; for one thing, coercion by health care workers is more likely to be practised and even advocated for in ways that would be anathema in the global north. While incentives may seem cheap or easy, caution is needed; and unlike something like a soda (offered in male circumcision in Kenya), the mama kits were needed for health and material well-being, and as such their use as an incentive should be approached with particular care.

*The Mama Kits as an Incentive or Reward*
*for Health Centre Delivery*

As I worked to tease out the rationale and use of the mama kits, another view was that the purpose of the mama kits was as an incentive or reward for giving birth in a health facility. Delivery care was less accessible than ANC, partly because of the nature of labour as a process whose timing cannot be planned and which impedes mobility. One could walk, bike, or be "doubled" by bicycle to ANC appointments; there was also some (albeit limited) flexibility in when to attend. For labour, a *boda-boda* (motorcycle taxi) was necessary and added to the expense and logistics of transportation. It was also necessary to bring an attendant, usually a co-wife, sister-in-law, or mother-in-law, increasing the cost of transportation. Marriage is generally patrilocal within Acholi communities (Baines & Rosenoff, 2014), hence the importance of in-laws. However, mothers of birthing women do also participate, as in the case of Jill, who told me about phoning her mother when her husband and mother-in-law were reluctant for her to spend money on a *boda* to deliver at the health centre, even though she had saved money by selling *mandazi* in the market. Her mother paid for the *boda*. Since health centres do not offer food or laundry services, patients need the assistance of a family member who will prepare food and wash clothes, as well as support the patient; these family members are referred to as attendants. Since cost depended on distance, those in the most remote households faced the highest costs in getting to a health facility for delivery. Birthing at home assisted by a TBA or a family member continued to be more common in remote places, especially when compared to practices in areas close to a fully operational health centre. This reflects access issues in the global south generally: "Poor geographic access has its greatest influence on the potential of women to reach a health facility during labour" (Munjanja et al., 2012, p. 146).

Florence described that she completed a full cycle of ANC, but she went on to say:

> It's the delivery that made me not to reach there [the health centre], I did not have money. Moving from here to Amuru needs money for transport ... so it's true that I gave birth from home.

She explained that her co-wives assisted at this difficult labour:

> The person who helped me? There wasn't anybody, but I was with my co-wives, and they are the ones who helped me. I began pushing the baby at 10 am and delivered at about 1 pm to 2 pm. I was in a very bad condition, but the child came out.

Participants who lived in remote villages where logistics including transportation impeded access to health centre delivery often related such stories of unplanned home births. Evidently because of the greater prevalence of home births in these remote villages, women there were less likely to have received a mama kit.

In the focus group held in Lujoro, a relatively remote town, four of the five participants had delivered at home. The fifth, Julia, gave birth on the way to the health centre; so of these five women, none had reached a health facility for delivery. The Lujoro group included a first-time mother and a mother of twins (who had been advised to deliver in a hospital); she spent the focus group tandem-nursing her babies as they spooned each other. The focus group situated in Pagak was, coincidentally, demographically similar; of the five women, one also happened to be a first-time mother and another the mother to recently born twins. All five women in Pagak, however, had given birth in the nearby health centre. This included one woman who was waiting at the health centre for an ambulance to take her to Lacor Hospital for a C-section when her baby arrived. The stark contrast between the near and far groups speaks to the influence of distance on access to care and illustrates how this structural factor supersedes a range of individual factors.

As I tried to understand the role of geography in accessing the mama kit, I asked Sophie, a 24-year-old with three children, whether mothers in her village (Oberabic) always received a mama kit. She confirmed, "When they have gone to the hospital [health centre], they get, but when you have given birth from home, you don't get." Indeed, I did not meet any mothers who had received mama kits after delivering at home or on the way to the health centre, even if they then brought their newborns for a check-up and immunization.

Because of the long distances to a functioning health centre and transportation difficulties, women sometimes gave birth on the way to a health facility, also rendering them ineligible for the mama kits. Children born on the way are often named Oyo or Ayo (the masculine and feminine forms) meaning "born on the way." Names associated with birth location, order, or position are common in Acholi culture, demonstrating the importance to families of how and where birth takes place. Julia from Lujoro gave birth on the way to the health centre. She went into labour and began to walk with her co-wives to the health centre and had just reached the turn off to the paved road (at Otwee) when her baby was born. She returned home, later going to the health centre for the baby's check-up and immunization. Ellen, who resided in Teddi, gave birth as she was returning home from her final ANC appointment, at which she had been told to come back if she was having labour pain. Because her home was such a long walk from the health centre, she spent the night at a halfway point. In the morning, labour came abruptly and she gave birth with the assistance of a stranger, naming her son Oyo. None of Ellen's 13 children had been born at a health centre. Ellen had lost seven children and had six living children. In my field notes, I record her apparent distress at not having been able to do more in relation to health care. However, this was the first pregnancy in which she had received ANC and HIV testing, perhaps an important milestone.

Jacky, from Teddi, was among the participants reporting that they did not receive a mama kit because they delivered elsewhere than a health centre. She said, "I did not get those gifts because when I delivered they should have taken me there [to the health centre], but because it was late they did not take me." Asked whether she was disappointed that she had not received the kit, she replied: "It did not disappoint me. I thought next time I would still get them." By "next time" she clarified that she meant the next time she had a baby. Such an attitude depended on women's ability to purchase the equivalent supplies themselves. Among women who had very little money, the mama kits were an especially valuable resource on which to depend.

Birthing at home or on the way meant women were denied a mama kit regardless of whether they had attended ANC. Jane, an 18-year-old first-time mother who had an older husband and one co-wife, told me that she had been unhappy to be pregnant and to (therefore) be compelled to marry. She had been afraid of giving birth. Jane had struggled to walk between her home in Teddi and ANC visits after the first visit, to which her husband had doubled her by bike. The walk was so long that she had to spend the night at a relative's home after each ANC visit. She wanted to go to the health centre to deliver as well, but the labour progressed quickly, such that her husband was concerned that she would give birth on the way if they tried to reach the health centre. The baby was, in fact, born before the TBA who they had called could arrive. Jane did not receive a mama kit when she took her baby to the health centre for a check-up following his birth. If the purpose of the kit was to reward compliance with ANC, as some posited, this woman "deserved" a kit. However, because she "failed" to deliver at a health centre, she was not eligible. In such situations, the mama kits held a punitive power over women who "chose" to give birth at home despite the health message that they should deliver at a health centre. For women like Jane or Jacky, birth location was determined by circumstances, including remote location, financial hardship, or precipitous labour, rather than by preference about birth location or type of birth attendant.

For Jane and Ellen's neighbour, Janet, the mama kits were part of what distinguished health centre delivery from home delivery. She had given birth to 11 children, all of whom were still living, remarkable in the context of high child mortality. During our interview, she sat with her seven-month-old daughter. Janet's first nine children had been born at home and the two most recent at the health centre. I asked her about the difference between giving birth at home and at the hospital. She said:

> Yes, there is some difference, as I saw with this child from the health centre. They gave some medicine for the eye, they gave soap, a bag, jelly, a basin, towels, and a pillow [case], which I saw as being different from the health centre as compared to the TBA. Also the delivery service at birth is different from the TBA, where they squeeze you for long to get the child out, while at the health centre they use some modern ways, and if they find that there is a difficulty they would then check up to know what could be the problem.

While Janet was aware of some clinical differences between the care at the health centre and that provided by TBAs, it was striking to me that the difference that first occurred to her was the provision of the mama kit supplies. Janet's most recent pregnancy had been very difficult, partly due to what she described as heart problems; she had been advised to avoid future pregnancy and said that she hoped to do so but did not have a clear plan.

### The Mama Kits as Supporting and Signalling "Vulnerable" Women

Despite the commonly held belief that the purpose of the mama kits was to incentivize the uptake of formal health care, many women also understood them as a form of economic support or help. For example, when I asked Margaret, a mother of five with one co-wife, why the mama kits were distributed, she said:

> The health centre has thought of helping mothers, that they should be helped, because some might be having a lot of problems and might not be able to buy those things, so they should be helped. Even if you will buy yours, that of the hospital should also be there.

It made sense to Margaret that mothers were offered some material assistance when having a baby, perhaps because of the post-conflict induced poverty, as well as experiences of humanitarian aid. Such an interpretation is supported by Hazel's suggestion, cited in chapter 3, that nutritionally enhanced foods distributed in the camps and during the initial return period should still be offered. Despite this view of the mama kits as providing material assistance for mothers, it was not the case that all mothers received mama kits.

I also heard about the kit as being targeted from Florence, who had been told that the mama kit was specifically for those with HIV. Knowing that I wanted to understand their purpose, she was emphatic:

> To me, they just told me, right to my face, that the [registration] card is for people who are HIV positive. That if you were positive, then they would register you when you are pregnant, but if you were healthy, then you would not be registered … She told me with her own mouth, that person registering.

As I later learned, understanding the mama kit as a form of assistance to mothers who were HIV positive accurately reflected one of the NGO's project goals. However, this was not a widespread understanding among childbearing women. Another resident of Lujoro, Rose, said she had learned the mama kit was for child mothers, older mothers, or mothers with disabilities. Outside of Lujoro, in the other five villages where I spoke with childbearing women, participants did not refer to the mama kits as a targeted program. Instead, most viewed them as a gift for new mothers and an incentive for health centre delivery.

Florence's response indicated her insight into the collusion of forces and discursive practices shaping maternity care and childbirth. She suggested that the most needed change was transportation between a nearby health centre where delivery care was unavailable and the functional health centre. In clarifying, she contrasted transportation with the mama kits:

> Yes, [a vehicle] that comes and gets people to take us there. But not like cloths or what, because those things will not help us. That's the help they give when they've seen how different you are. But what connects us [i.e., transportation] should at least be there.

For her, facilitating access to care was more important than the material goods offered via the mama kits. She identified that the mama kits operated as a strategy of difference but advocated for an intervention that would directly facilitate access. Such an interpretation is also supported in a discussion of gifts in development that makes the case that "gifts, like charity, do not lead to easy identification but, rather, to a reaffirmation of difference" (Stirrat & Henkel, 1997, p. 80). In Amuru, NGOs were often associated with Westerners or non-community members: for this participant, the mama kits re-inscribed the differences, including wealth and poverty, between those supplying and those receiving NGO resources. While marking local women's poverty and lack of access to basic supplies, the mama kits had little capacity to address the causes of this poverty or to significantly intervene in women's circumstances. Strikingly, Florence referred to transportation as "what connects us," suggesting that the priority should be on tangible means of reaching care, rather than token support. In the absence of help that could facilitate access to care in a practical manner, she rejected the idea of "cloths or what," as offered in the mama kits.

A number of participants critiqued vulnerability as an impractical and divisive criteria, leading me to reflect on the nature of vulnerability as a discursive category within global health interventions. In a practical sense, the majority of pregnant Acholi women I encountered were materially vulnerable, in that they needed support beyond what was immediately available to them in their everyday lives. This vulnerability is a consequence of political events and social norms and structures yet becomes located in their bodies and stories. Academic feminists have also worked to explore the limits of vulnerability discourse and the ways in which it is paired with particular groups of women and with particular places. Judith Butler (2015) suggests that while vulnerability can constitute an empirical sociological observation, when it becomes a "new norm of description" it can reproduce the pattern in which it was previously working to intervene (p. 139). Erinn Gilson suggests that to avoid a reductive view of vulnerability, it is best understood as "a process rather than as a quasi-fixed property of places and people" (2018, p. 232). While vulnerability is a convenient shorthand for workers in service-providing NGOs, this framing is not without its consequences.

### The Mama Kits as a Gift or Charity

Despite recognizing that the mama kits play a role as an incentive to access care, for childbearing women participants, the primary utility of the kits was for the material goods to help with the new baby. These were some of the same goods for which women took on additional jobs, such as selling snacks or ploughing a neighbour's field. Women referred to the mama kits as a gift,[1] for example, by saying, "I came back without any gift" or "there are some gifts that they give you from there [health centre]." This language calls to mind Mauss's work on gift exchange in which gifts are freely given yet also create a social obligation for some form of reciprocity.

--------

1 The Acholi word is *mic.*

In this case, the obligation could be seen as the requirement to comply with care. Other forms of giving in this setting, particularly prominent during the later years of the conflict, are charity and humanitarian aid. Aid can be construed as different from a gift in being offered altruistically, without the expectation of reciprocity (Zarowsky, 2000). Familiar with humanitarian aid delivered in the IDP camps on the basis of need and suffering, childbearing women continued to foreground their need for material goods when interpreting this new "gift," the goals of which appear to be developmental rather than humanitarian. This exemplifies a disjuncture between childbearing participants' understanding of the gift as useful and necessary – typified by a participant's suggestion that as well as cloths, there should be "clothes for wearing, a jumper for the cold" – and the extra-local attempts to use the gift as a means to promote skilled attendance at birth and knowledge of ANC.

Receiving or not receiving care is not abstract to recipients; it signals important messages about inclusion and belonging and has real material impacts. For recipients of NGO project goods, "what starts off as an anonymous abstract donation becomes personalized and concretized" (Stirrat & Henkel, 1997, p. 77). This is evident in participants' feelings – including blame, envy, and frustration – about being passed over for the gift. For example, Lily pointed to an equity issue, telling me, "Those things that your friends get, if they are there [i.e., exist], then the help should be for everyone." In this, as in other international development projects, community members who do not benefit from a project nevertheless have to organize their lives in relation to the project. Orienting to the position of people in recipient communities like Amuru, Krause (2014) writes, "We have to consider that only a small share of those who might be said to need help actually receive help, that there is thus a competition among gift receivers but that those who do not receive also give" (p. 58). Navigating potential gifts can become part of the health work of being pregnant. While relief helps its recipients, "recipients also give something in return: consent, time, and labor … They give this labor under conditions over which they have very little control" (Krause, 2014, p. 60). Competition, work, embodying difference, and detracting from practical solutions are some negative effects of the mama kit project for childbearing women in Amuru sub-county, who nevertheless both need and want the material goods distributed via the project.

### Registration and Distribution of Mama Kits

The registration and distribution of the mama kits was a topic of concern for participants, as it was neither straightforward nor predictable.

To receive the kit, women were required to have a registration card, distinct from the ANC card. Registration cards were white or yellow with a Red Cross logo and were given to expectant women by a VHT member. The pregnant woman's name was recorded in a registration book, so that health centre staff distributing the kits could cross-refer. The requirement to register occurred in addition to any other actual or perceived requirements for receiving the mama kits, such as attending ANC or giving birth at the health centre. Registration took place as outreach, in which case the VHT member would visit households, or on a given day at the health centre, in which case women would be informed that their local VHT representative would register people, say, every Thursday at the health centre.

The mama kit registration card functioned as an IE text in that by receiving these cards, women were being brought into a form of social organization that relied on extra-local bureaucracies, discourses, and goals. In this case, the Red Cross programming and its implementation of global health goals were an extra-local force; to receive the mama kits, women had to meet the standards required to get the registration cards and the mama kits. When registration was routine, it meant women were coordinating their care around the requirements they saw as necessary to be registered and to receive the kits. When the process of registration failed or excluded women, it left them without access to the mama kits, a resource they felt entitled to and were frustrated not to receive.

Participants described the process of receiving a registration card for the mama kits as complicated. One mother did not receive a card but nevertheless received a mama kit:

> I didn't get that card in my hand. I was told if you go for ANC four times you receive the card, but I didn't receive [it], even after we were told they [the VHT] would come here and give us it. So I went [to ANC] four times and they stopped me. I went and stayed home only for three days and delivered at hospital [health centre]. I had to go back home, because that day there was no immunization, because they were immunizing within villages for a week [i.e., the health centre was understaffed due to outreach], so I went back after they had called us. Then we were given the white card [mama kit registration card] but the person in charge said their home was far behind Otwee so they distributed the things and collected back the card. So they gave us a bag, soap, baby clothes, and one carrier.

This woman's persistence and the initial work she had put into complying with ANC attendance paid off. Her story demonstrated the unpredictable work involved in trying to link to the system of the card and the mama kit.

Other participants who were not registered during pregnancy were less fortunate and did not receive a kit. For example, Isla from Rec Kicere shared:

> I have heard about that gift, but the person in charge of registering here is up to Mutema [a remote village] while others stay at the hospital [health centre], so we in Rec Kicere are to be registered in Mutema, the lady does not like being at the hospital [health centre].

Or, on a similar note, Beryl did not get registered or get a mama kit:

> Whenever I went to the hospital [health centre], they would tell us that registration is always on Thursdays and if we went on Thursday we would find those who register from the local village around. But [a VHT member] from our side would not be around.

In such circumstances, participants did not know where to turn and had to give up on receiving a mama kit.

In half of the villages where I conducted interviews, the women identified the registration problem as stemming from specific VHT members. In two neighbouring villages, the VHT member lived in a remote part of their area, possibly making outreach for registration difficult for her. In the third village, the VHT member responsible for registering pregnant women had moved and had not been replaced. It was in the most remote villages where many women experienced barriers to registration and did not receive the mama kits. In these villages, giving birth at home, sometimes with a TBA attending, was also more prevalent. If the mama kits were intended as an incentive, they might have been expected to have the most impact in such areas; however, it was in remote areas that access to the kit was most problematic. Participants said the particular VHT member, Justine, did not like to travel to register people or to go to the health centre to meet women and register them. This would have been a considerable distance for her to travel likely at some expense. Further, some participants mentioned that the VHT member herself had a small baby, which might be keeping her close to home. While it is possible that the registration problem stemmed from this VHT member's unwillingness or inability to register women, there is also another possibility. One health worker explained to me that each VHT member was given a limited number of registration cards (to correspond with the limited number of mama kits available). Justine might have used up her supply of cards, and therefore stopped registering people. Limited provision of the mama kits and registration cards meant that their registration and distribution regulated women's activities in relation to maternity care.

This scarcity of registration cards and kits created inequitable access. Inequalities in access to the basic supplies necessary to care for a newborn are structured by power relationships; such inequalities are not simply a problem of resource supply and/or allocation. Scarcity can be understood as a discourse, one that, as Ingram (2013) writes,

> pathologizes the poor while diverting attention away from questions of inequality and distribution. In a climate of austerity, the neoliberal discourse of scarcity risks complicity with a politics of abandonment. (p. 450)

This analysis fits the circumstances under which scarcity was invoked in relation to mama kits for women in Amuru. The items women received in the mama kits were valuable for their practical use. These items could neither substantially alleviate poverty nor significantly impact maternal-child health issues. Yet in the context of constrained access to material goods and the reproduction of scarcity via policies governing their access, the kits became something women worked for and organized their care around.

The problems with the mechanisms of registration and distribution of the mama kits were located in the inequitable power arrangements between childbearing women, the VHT, health centre staff, and the NGOs. Tracing the texts involved in registration and the sequences of activities it coordinated allowed me a view into how extra-local activities and priorities influenced activities and priorities at the local level. The activities of the local middle-people (the VHT and health centre staff) were constrained by professional organization. For example, the Red Cross initially identified VHT members responsible for registering women for the mama kits. However, when individual VHT members' capacity to perform this task changed, the Red Cross was not locally present to re-appoint someone (focus group in Pagak; Peter, June 28, 2012). Based elsewhere, NGO work had little continuity within Amuru. The DHO and the clinical officer in-charge of the health centre, to their frustration, had limited control over the organization and scope of the mama kits project. This form of NGO involvement, however, shaped the way the health district and health centre provided care. For local health workers, their capacity to deliver care was organized within parameters defined by outside forces. Discourses of scarcity and deservedness contributed to how these parameters were defined.

## Health Centre Staff and Administrators on the Mama Kits' Role: Helping the Vulnerable or Incentivizing Compliance?

I spoke with health workers, as well as mothers, about the role of the mama kits. Health centre administrators and staff differed in their understandings of the mama kits' purpose. Those with an administrative role identified two purposes: one stated by the donor organization – providing assistance to vulnerable women – and one developed through local practices – providing an incentive or reward to those women who completed ANC and delivered in the hospital. Front line staff, who worked directly with pregnant and birthing women, spoke only of the second purpose, perhaps demonstrating their acceptance of the way the gift had been instrumentalized. However, their use of the mama kits as an incentive was acknowledged and encouraged by the clinical officer in charge, Jonas, who administered the health centre.

### "In Our Setting, Who Is the Most Poor?" Perceptions of Vulnerability as a Distribution Criteria

The two health care administrator participants, Jonas and Peter, were the clinical officer in-charge at Lacor HCIII and the DHO, respectively. The most senior health worker at the health centre, Jonas was both the manager and a clinician. Jonas was a neighbour who, like me, lived in staff housing located just above the health centre; he acted as a host in helping my family get situated, and we spoke often and at length about health care delivery, in addition to the interview that I recorded. Peter was a government employee overseeing health services in Amuru district, in which Amuru sub-county is situated; a dentist by training, his work in Amuru was in senior government administration. Peter lived in neighbouring Gulu, he and his wife commuting long distances in opposite directions for their work while, as with Jonas's, his children studied at boarding school. Jonas answered my question about whether or not the mama kits project was universal by stating, "[Who receives one is] selective, yeah, the ones who have been identified and seen that they really need these." However, as he later described, selection criteria were neither clearly articulated nor followed. Peter had a similar view about how need was determined: "Yes, … that was why I said they should expand it, they were targeting the most vulnerable … the most poor. But in our setting here, who is the most poor?" In the context of widespread poverty, a targeted project in which the resource distribution takes place under an ideology and a practice of scarcity makes distribution competitive and inequitable. Peter also highlighted the fact that despite his senior role as DHO, it was external NGO actors, and not government health officers, who controlled how the mama kits were deployed to childbearing women.

The responses of the health administrators demonstrate problems with "vulnerability" as a distribution criterion. In a setting of widespread poverty and poor infrastructure, it was difficult and counterproductive to determine who was most vulnerable. Further, this type of intervention does little to address the inequities that increase such vulnerabilities.

An additional problem with vulnerability as a distribution criterion was that it limited supplies, such that shortages resulted when those distributing the mama kits tried to use their own criteria, such as whether birth took place at a health facility. When I asked him about distribution, Peter acknowledged inconsistencies and lack of clarity surrounding the project goal of assisting vulnerable women, and the difficulty identifying those women most deserving of the mama kits:

> The concept of the project was to help the vulnerable women, those women who fear to come to the health facility because they cannot buy the plastic sheeting, they have no soap, they have no baby clothes. It was primarily to remove that barrier. But you see, everybody needs those things, and they have a big challenge, who to give, who to not give. And I think they almost give to everyone. The VHTs are supposed to have been the ones to sort out: "You, you are in a better situation, you should not. Let another woman who is in a worse off situation than you get it." But of course it is not easy.

The sheeting Peter refers to is a length of heavy black plastic to be used as a bed cover, in order to prevent cross-contamination of the delivery bed. The midwives sometimes sat together on their stoop chatting and cutting these from a longer length, selling them as a side business. Each woman was required to bring her own plastic sheeting at the time of delivery; it was something women saved for as a delivery expense. The poor were not a subgroup; rather, the population at large was experiencing poverty in the aftermath of war. Asked by an NGO representative to assess the mama kit program, Peter had spoken of its positive impact and requested that it be expanded. But despite Peter's responsibility for health in the district as DHO, the NGOs' operations ultimately placed the decision outside his jurisdiction and that of frontline health workers. When NGO programming shapes care provision, but health care providers can't make decisions about NGO programming, the autonomy and capability of health care providers to best meet their patient needs is threatened.

### Health Centre Staff on the Mama Kit: "Motivating" Women to Deliver at a Health Facility

While acknowledging that the NGOs intended the mama kit program to intervene in situations where women were vulnerable, both Jonas and Peter saw the kits as a useful means by which to create an incentive for attending health centres. Jonas summarized this as follows: "So these women who live very far now tend to say, 'Okay, since I have been registered, let me go and deliver there and I get these items, because if I deliver from home I will miss these items.'" Similarly, Peter stated, "That small thing really helps women come [to the health facility]." While it is clear that addressing systemic barriers would have the greatest impact, Peter's perspective that providing an incentive can play a role in promoting skilled delivery is corroborated by a study finding that "provision of free delivery kits to mothers who delivered at the health facility significantly increased skilled attended delivery" (Ediau et al., 2013, p. 19) in Kitgum, a northern Uganda town, during a study in which the kit was introduced as an incentive. The impact of such an incentive was, however, found to be limited in a study by Mbonye and colleagues (2013) who tracked the results of a "motivation project," which included a version of the mama kit, as well as education in improving the rates of adherence to malaria prevention and facility delivery in another area of Uganda. They found that this motivation package did improve adherence but acknowledged that "despite this, relatively few women delivered at health facilities. Constraints like high costs, long distances to health facilities and the role of the husband could have influenced this outcome" (Mbonye et al., 2013, p. 6). Inevitably, in the absence of adequate access to care, incentivizing care seeking has limited impact. It also, as I argue here, can shift attention away from the systemic changes required and towards the behaviours or decisions of individual women, responsibilizing individuals for poor outcomes that in reality are a problem of a neglected health system and its limited reach.

Peter claimed that while the mama kit, or gift, was small, it was helpful and perhaps necessary: "They need those mama kits! They cannot afford it. And even if you have saved some money and you can afford, it is not there!" His phrase "not there" introduces a common Acholi expression into English meaning not present, non-existent, and refers to the fact that most people did not live near shops that sold cloths, basins, or baby jelly. As with the mother participants in the study's first phase, Peter saw the kits as necessary and useful. Together, Peter and Jonas leveraged the kits' utility to create incentives to participate in health care.

Health workers caring directly for birthing women (those who did not have an administrative role or much interaction with NGO staff) saw the purpose of the mama kits primarily as an incentive or a reward and not as providing resources to vulnerable women. This excerpt from my interview with Amy, the nursing assistant, was typical. She begins by recapping my question:

> Why they give them, eh? Motivation is why. Just to motivate them. (Sarah): Motivation to deliver here? (Amy): Eh [agreement]. Because they give that [those] things just simply for those ones who come to deliver in the hospital. And for you, if you want that mama kit, you should make sure you come and deliver in the hospital.

Other staff used terms like "a morale booster" (the public health educator, William), "encouragement" (William, midwife Grace, nurse Nancy), and "to motivate" (midwife Gloria, Amy, above). Grace clarified that the reason for such encouragement was the goal of reducing maternal and infant mortality through an increase in health centre birth. She said, "The main reason, eh? In order to encourage the mother to deliver in the hospital [health centre]. By that it will reduce maternal and child what? Death. That is the main purpose." The midwives repeatedly spoke about avoiding maternal and infant death, a dominant discourse shaping their work and an issue of critical concern.

### The Goals of the Uganda Red Cross

To clarify the mama kits project's goals, I contacted Red Cross Uganda. I learned that the goal of the Safe Motherhood Project, as it is called, was that "pregnant women in Amuru and Kitgum district give birth safely under the sanitary environment" and "to contribute to the increase in health centre delivery and antenatal care attendance up to four times by pregnant mothers." The project activities were described as follows: "Register vulnerable pregnant women who would be supported by this project. Procure and distribute mama kits per year to vulnerable pregnant women. Procure and distribute essential sanitary materials and delivery equipment to health center" (unpublished document, A. Onzima, Uganda Red Cross, March 10, 2014).

Based on these objectives, operating as an incentive to ANC and particularly delivery care was in keeping with the project's goals. *Vulnerability* was not defined in the document that outlined the project goals, perhaps contributing to the ambiguity regarding how the kits should be allocated (personal communication, A. Onzima, Uganda Red Cross, March 10, 2014). The project did not appear to take into account women's different social and geographic locations with regard to delivery care access. Similarly, while suggesting that women would be "supported" by the project, a consideration of the extent or limitations of such support was absent. All stakeholders shared a broad concern over maternal health; however, in other instances, the lack of shared concerns was evident in the different ways "vulnerability" or "support" were operationalized.

## NGO–Health Centre Partnerships: Problems with Withdrawal and Shortages

With NGO projects, program closures and supply shortages are a constant threat. Several senior staff members raised the issue of closure. The clinical officer in-charge, Jonas, framed his concerns in reference to a previous Northern Uganda Malaria Aids and Tuberculosis (NUMAT) project, which he introduced as an analogous situation: "These mosquito nets we used to distribute during antenatal clinic, and then the mama kits we would give at delivery. And this one ended because the program also ended." While distributing the mosquito nets was part of the ANC goal to reduce the incidence of malaria among pregnant women (a major cause of infant death), it was not a health centre initiative but an NGO initiative. Its sustainability, as Jonas described, was beyond the control of the health centre.

When asked about the mama kit, Peter, like Jonas, raised the closure of the NUMAT program, which had offered sleeping nets and something similar to the mama kit, as an illustrative example. He pointed out that the transitory nature of program support was typical. He began by saying it had increased women's attendance at health centres:

> So because of that they will come in big numbers, and it was something really the government will provide, they were providing, but you know our government. Things are not ... they usually end, even if the idea is very good, somewhere the idea breaks.

In the case of mama kits, the government supply chain did have kits available for purchase, but their cost and the high number of births made purchasing the kits impractical (Jonas). The government's failure to provide free kits to health centres led to a situation in which health centres were willing to collaborate with NGOs and international NGOs out of need, a reliance on donor projects that has typified Uganda's approach to health intervention (Whyte et al., 2013, p. 155). However, such collaborations were noted to be unsustainable. The withdrawal of NGOs, or closure of particular NGO programs, is something that health workers anticipate but cannot plan for. As the public health educator, Alex, explained, "So you know, with the Red Cross, they may withdraw, if they find that their work is needed somewhere else." Inherent in the structure of health centres delivering NGO projects alongside clinical care is a lack of control and certainty. Such unpredictability was one of the negative consequences of NGO interventions in maternal health. When projects on which women rely end or have limited reach, this contributes to the fragility of the health system rather than bolstering it.

With the war over and resettlement well underway, many NGO programs had moved on, such that NGO withdrawal was a particular feature of Amuru and post-conflict northern Uganda. In a study of early childhood in the transition period following conflict, the problem of rapid NGO withdrawal was described and the case made that "a gradual withdrawal of services that is responsive to the rate of transition" would be preferable to rapid withdrawal of services on which people still depend (McElroy, 2012, p. 147). If the mama kits project were to stop, the health centre staff would seek new strategies to provide resources or incentives, and childbearing women would be left without this support.

In addition to the problem of NGO withdrawal shaping health care delivery, health care providers faced the challenge of managing the stock of the mama kit. As Jonas described it, the number of kits supplied was too low, because the large area and population served by Lacor HCIII was not taken into consideration; instead, all health centres received the same number of kits without regard to the numbers of deliveries. As Jonas pointed out, "They [NGOs] do their calculation uniformly, with all the other health facilities in the other sub-counties, not knowing that other sub-counties have like two HCIIIs or one HCIII plus three or four HCIIs that are well functioning." Jonas indicated this left him and his staff in the position of having to explain to mothers when the mama kits ran out. The large number of births at Lacor HCIII was shaped by lack of capacity in neighbouring health centres.

One strategy for managing the limited supply was to divide the kits, which partly accounted for the discrepancies participants reported in what they received. Jonas explained:

The Red Cross provides mama bags with a basin, a baby gel, two towels, a dress for the baby. That is what is in the bag, then outside the bag they have a piece of bathing soap, and we give them two bars of soap. Sometimes when the bags are few we give them one-one [i.e., the contents of the kit are divided].

This strategy stretched supplies, to come closer to being able to offer one at each health centre birth, but contributed to the confusion over what women received. Similarly, when they had supplies, the health centre staff sometimes gave bars of soap to husbands who had attended ANC and tested for HIV, to encourage this practice. The role of male partner HIV testing is discussed further in chapter 5. Dividing the kits in these ways may have accounted for one participant who had received most items in the kit but who complained that a staff member had stolen the soap. Using limited resources to leverage or promote a wide range of health efforts contributed to their scarcity and the effects of that scarcity.

The mama kit was an intervention from the "outside," introduced by national and international NGOs, and carried with it these outside agencies' beliefs and discourses about the experiences and needs of local women. For example, the attempt to identify and assist vulnerable individuals was not acceptable to childbearing women or health workers, despite the prominence of vulnerability as a criterion on which humanitarian and development interventions are based. While people were differentially socially located, all families were willing to organize their activities around receiving the kit, since they valued its goods and regarded them as useful. Health administrators and workers had discarded aspects of the program that they had discerned as having little local relevance (such as identifying especially vulnerable women). Health workers who delivered the program adapted it to support their own goals; in particular, increasing the number of women attending ANC and delivering in a health care facility. While this was a valuable goal, the mama kits did not address the primary reasons that women do not access care.

Health workers' adaptations of the mama kits project to their own professional goals were creative and resourceful, yet they acted as a coercive measure to leverage pregnant women's material need as a means of getting them to attend health centre care. At the same time, the need for creative adaptation indicated a mismatch between health centre and NGO goals. This mismatch, and lack of health centre authority in delivering the NGOs' project, caused problems for the adapted version of the mama kits project. For example, when creatively reinterpreted as a more universal program for those attending ANC and delivering in a facility, a shortfall occurred. As I argue below, when registration cards or kits ran out, women hoping to receive this "gift" saw the process as arbitrary. These negative consequences of the mama kits project indicated a discordant vision between NGOs such as the Red Cross and other stake-holders including health providers and clients. This was exacerbated by inequities in these relationships.

The problems for health providers working with NGOs, including a lack of overlap in goals, instability, lack of continuity, and lack of autonomy on the local partners delivering the project, are widespread. Pfeiffer and Nichter (2008) assert:

> We are concerned by reports of wasteful spending, poor planning, and uncoordinated project development, which suggest a growing anarchy on the ground in global health efforts. This state of anarchy is fueled by an avalanche of resources landing on neglected health systems facing work-force shortages and crumbling infrastructure unprepared to manage this largesse. (pp. 410–411)

The mama kits, taken together with other products and projects of NGOs, such as mosquito nets, therapeutic feeding products, and others, demand significant resources and staff time.[2] It is even more significant when one considers that the project has been taking place at a time when there was one doctor practising in Amuru district, a district of approximately 190,516 people in 2014 (Republic of Uganda, 2015), and when the government health centre has been operating without any beds in the labour room, to the protest of local parturient women.

## Unpredictable Distribution Affects How Women Perceive Formal Care and Health Workers

Variance in whether women received a kit, when they received it, and what it included, coloured women's perceptions of health workers. It appeared to participants that health workers had the power to arbitrarily determine how and to whom supplies would be allocated. This reinforced a dynamic of the health centre as a site of difference and power. Participants said that receiving a kit depended on the following: luck; possession of an appropriate registration card; the location of the birth; women's HIV status; whether or not staff were overtired; and/or the availability of supplies. Participants thus viewed the kits themselves

---

2  In my field notes, I wrote a single line on May 23: "Someone at [my son's] school had *Plumpy'nut* as their school snack today." Later on, I wrote, "The kids (of the health centre staff) are snacking on *Plumpy'nut* today (the sachets for therapeutic feeding for malnourished children). That's got to be a frustration for the WHO or whoever supplies these" (July 2012).

in positive terms but had less positive accounts of their distribution. Lack of transparency eroded the trust and common ground between birthing women and health facilities or staff, leading to an alienating effect. A similar pattern was found in a study of perceptions of care quality among mothers and health workers in Mpigi and Rukungiri districts (Uganda); when health workers developed "informal solutions" because of structural problems in the health system, it led to "mistrust, inequity in care and negative experiences" (Munabi-Babigumira et al., 2019, p. 13).

For example, Beryl, an Alur woman who had moved at age 14 to Teddi in Amuru from the West Nile area to be with her husband and was now a 23-year-old mother of three, found the unevenness and unpredictability of distribution frustrating:

> That friend of mine who is wearing the *kitenge* [African fabric] blouse registered together with me because we live together. She was given a gift and I wasn't given … I was so hurt. And yet my friends are getting, and my name was registered, then they did not give me … I was so annoyed.

The inequity of being excluded was unsettling.

One of the two midwives working at Lacor HCIII, Gloria, acknowledged that women could experience the health centre as somewhere they were judged or discriminated against. In response to a question about misunderstandings that maternity care recipients had, she said, "They don't want to give them [the mama kits], they think, 'there, they segregate people. They give [the mama kit] to others, they don't give to others,' not knowing what the reason is." Gloria saw this as a misunderstanding that affected care, whereas birthing women found the unpredictability frustrating or unfair. Unknown criteria in the distribution of mama kits led to differences in how women encountered health centre care; Gloria saw this as contributing to a negative perception of the health centre and its staff.

## Conclusion

The mama kits project provides a window into translocal aspects of the organization of maternity care and birth in Amuru sub-county through which we can see how the goals and values of extra-local groups and local people competed. While participants wanted and appreciated the mama kits, the kits were supplied within the context of a neglected and an inadequate health system and were used to coerce women's care-seeking practices, albeit within a difficult context in which high maternal mortality led health workers to improvise strategies to increase the number of health centre deliveries. When considered within the overall approach to maternity care, the layering of a marginal form of social support onto a dysfunctional health system can be seen as governing through scarce resources in this marginalized region. Such an approach contributed to the ongoing pathologizing of poverty (Farmer, 2008, p. 2010). As Pfeiffer and Nichter (2008) explain, "There is a growing recognition of the urgent need to build or rebuild health systems, yet the increasing flow of aid from donors continues to promote narrow interventions and specific projects. This 'stove-piping' of projects creates additional stress on government health infrastructures while providing little in the way of institution building" (p. 411). In drawing on considerable resources while not contributing to the development of the health care system, the mama kit exemplifies such a project. Access to care, coercive power, and translocal goals are themes that are also evident in practices surrounding couples' HIV testing during ANC, discussed in the next chapter.

# Chapter Five

# Vertical Health: Failures of Compulsory Couples' HIV Testing

## Introduction

In this chapter, I trace a compulsory and coercive approach to couples' HIV testing during ANC and identify its negative impacts on gender relations and on health care. The coercive approach to testing in northern Uganda conflicted with both national policies and international approaches, yet stemmed from local efforts to comply with both. Compulsory testing is not identified in global health approaches governing maternity care or HIV prevention and indeed contravenes global health rhetoric around rights and access. This kind of policy misapplication, however, is encouraged by key features of conventional global health practices, including a vertical approach and a standardized approach. Where a horizontal approach addresses multiple challenges simultaneously by broadly targeting health systems, a vertical approach addresses health issues one at a time in stand-alone silos. Within a standardized approach, context-specific economic and social factors tend to be neglected in favour of a one-size-fits-all solution. Here, I track how global health goals related to HIV prevention were mistranslated in the practice of maternity care in Amuru, to help elucidate the shortcomings of a vertical, standardized approach to global health challenges.

The goal of preventing HIV transmission during pregnancy and childbirth shapes maternity care in Amuru sub-county, as elsewhere. The testing of pregnant women and their partners during ANC, known as couples' testing, was widely perceived by expectant mothers to be compulsory and indeed was presented as such by health centre staff. A compulsory approach to HIV testing during ANC impacts the rights and lives of women and men, with inequitable gender and power relationships exacerbating the negative impacts of such an approach. These negative impacts on women included additional work in accessing care, potential intimate partner violence, and increased barriers to ANC and delivery care as I have described in an earlier gender relations analysis of testing practices (Rudrum et al., 2017). Practices were coercive to pregnant women, burdening them with the task of facilitating male involvement and making future ANC and delivery care contingent on their ability to recruit their husbands to participate. Testing practices contributed to a shift in role in which health workers, expected to police testing, act as gatekeepers to delivery care and were thereby pulled away from a focus on providing care. While such gendered dynamics impacting care tend to be seen through a lens focused on local culture, what stands out to me is the ways in which they are, in fact, substantially shaped by relatively distal factors, including international decisions governing global health.

## Background: Prevalence, Policies, and Practice

Despite being known for its early successes in HIV prevention, Uganda has the 10th-highest HIV prevalence in the world at 7.3 per cent (adult prevalence; Uganda Bureau of Statistics, 2011). The highest-prevalence countries are all in sub-Saharan Africa, with three countries facing rates over 20 per cent, dramatically higher than Uganda's. Within the context of the HIV epidemic on the continent, Uganda was once lauded as a success story for its early interventions in stemming transmission rates, but this success is now a thing of the past as rates begin to rise in some parts of the country (Hladik, 2008; Parkhurst, 2011; Shafer et al., 2008). This is reflected in national rates, while the upheaval caused by recent conflict and displacement has contributed to higher rates of HIV in northern Uganda, perhaps double the prevalence in the country as a whole (Westerhaus et al., 2007). (An increase to HIV rates is not always the case in conflict settings, as discussed by Adia Benton in her book *HIV Exceptionalism: Development Through Disease in Sierra Leone*, 2015.) Rates among pregnant women in the north of Uganda are high – 11.3 per cent among women accessing ANC at a major hospital – a pattern attributed to "social and economic crises, food shortages, population displacement and reduced access to health care" resulting from the conflict (Fabiani et al., 2006, p. 590). The rates measured at ANC are sometimes used as a proxy measure for the general population, as it is a widespread site of surveillance (Chan, 2015, p. 30; Walker et al., 2003, p. 2219). This form of sentinel surveillance is useful but never fully accurate as it introduces biases (Eaton et al., 2014, p. S513; Zaba et al., 2000). No rate is available for Amuru district; however, in neighbouring Gulu district, 12.8 per cent of young adults are HIV positive (Patel et al., 2014b).

Throughout Africa, heterosexual sex is the most common mode of HIV transmission, with the vertical transmission to babies a parallel epidemic. Women are disproportionately affected by the virus (Padian et al., 2011;

Wawer et al., 2009), as well as bearing a greater disease burden than men, and young women (15 to 24) are "more than twice as likely to become newly infected with HIV as men the same age" (Sia et al., 2014, p. 939).

While an HIV test for pregnant women is recommended in most settings, in places with high HIV prevalence, like Uganda, the testing of both partners in a couple is promoted to prevent mother-to-child transmission (PMTCT), also referred to as vertical transmission. Transmission can occur during pregnancy, birth, or breastfeeding, but is preventable via the use of antiretroviral drugs, making testing an important element of prevention. The risk to the infant can best be understood in the context of the HIV status of both parents, rather than solely the mother's status, since an HIV-positive partner may transmit the virus to the mother during pregnancy. Throughout Uganda, couples' testing is offered at the first ANC visit, one of four appointments during focused ANC. An important feature of ANC is the antenatal card, which is issued to women and details health information pertinent to their pregnancy, delivery, and postnatal care. Once identified, a woman's HIV status is recorded on her ANC card, as is that of her husband if available. However, this relies on the husband's attendance at this appointment and his willing participation. Thus, testing can be impeded by social norms of maternity care as an arena solely for women and by men's reluctance to test, among other challenges.

National policy at the time of research identified couples' testing as a routine and provider-initiated health care service from which patients could opt out. Intended to boost the number of people being tested, the routine, provider-initiated approach departed from the voluntary counselling and testing approach of the 1990s, which reflected human rights discourses (Vernooij & Hardon, 2013). More recently, the approach to testing has changed again as a result of the *HIV and AIDS Prevention and Control Act, 2014* (Republic of Uganda, 2014), which makes testing compulsory ("routine" as opposed to "voluntary") for pregnant women and their partners. What I observed, however, and what I learned from speaking with pregnant women and their care providers, was that couples' testing was implemented within Amuru in such a way that it was believed to be compulsory well in advance of this policy change.

*A Compulsory Approach in Amuru*

In Amuru sub-county, women and their husbands were instructed to attend the first ANC appointment together, according to both childbearing women and health worker participants. I observed this message when accompanying staff during outreach visits to villages, as well as in the public health talks offered to patients in the waiting room, before the health centre opened each morning. Prominent public signs and posters also exhorted men to accompany their partners to ANC. Large metal signs at the turnoffs to health centres read "If you love your wife, then go together with her to the hospital when she is pregnant." I took pictures in the outpatient ward of a poster showing a man doubling a pregnant woman on a bicycle, with the caption "Responsible men go early with their wives for antenatal care. Test today together with your wife for HIV so that you prevent transmission of the virus to the unborn baby still in the womb."

These signs and posters call on men to be responsible, honest, and loving citizens, messaging that attempts to appeal to masculine ideals of men as protectors or providers. However, it was their pregnant partners who were called on to persuade men to attend. This shifting of responsibility to individuals and away from systems as a feature of neoliberal health care is an example of responsibilization. The strategy of requiring women to be responsible for men's participation in testing and ANC disregarded the reluctance men often expressed and the difficulty women therefore had in bringing a partner. Moreover, positioning women as responsible for the health of the family reified gendered divisions of the labour of care.

*Women's Experiences of Male Reluctance*

It was through participants that I learned about the couples' test as a difficult moment in ANC, one that impacted their future care. Women's accounts of their partners' reluctance to test and to attend ANC helped me to understand the impacts of a coercive approach to couples' testing. Women who encountered resistance from their male partners attributed it to the view that pregnancy was a woman's concern and to fear over HIV status. This view of pregnancy as a women-only issue was mentioned to me many times in a wide range of contexts, indicating, perhaps, not only its prominence but also its contested nature. While sharing with me, my RA, and four other participants during a focus group, Anne situated male reluctance to attend ANC within male apathy towards women's lives during pregnancy:

> When you tell some men to go together with you to the hospital, he doesn't accept. You can force him, but he will still refuse. Then you get your own way of going alone to get a card … If you don't go for a check-up yourself he doesn't care. He just sits. Women just struggle for themselves alone.

During another focus group, as one woman was complaining that her husband did nothing to help during pregnancy, another member pointed out "he's right there!" – he was walking by the shade tree where we were sitting. She was unconcerned, stating that it was a fact: he did nothing. Sara, from Rec Kicere, said that her husband had agreed to attend ANC during her second and most recent pregnancy but had refused during her first pregnancy. She recalled his position that "nothing takes me to the hospital." He had argued that since he wasn't sick, there was no point in testing. She believed, however, that in fact he feared he *did* have the virus and that "he would rather not know." Other participants also said their husbands feared the lifestyle changes that would accompany a positive status, including the difficulty of "wooing" other women.

Both childbearing women and health worker participants speculated that in addition to fear of the virus and wanting to distance themselves from "women's matters," men had sometimes already independently tested positive and did not want to disclose their status. For example, Faith, a focus group participant in Pagak said, "There are men when they already know their status as positive, they will not want to be supported by hospital. Some may start to go [for ANC and HIV testing], but nearing the hospital they disappear." Several participants recounted this problem of men disappearing at the last minute. Alcohol use was another form of avoidance. Inexpensive *waragi*, a strong clear alcohol, was available in small plastic sachets (since banned); these could be found discarded along public paths. Penny compared alcohol dependence to a contract, something difficult to break: "Alcohol is a difficult issue to handle, because even if you stop a man he will not listen. Alcohol is just like a contract that people have signed."

Despite such difficulties, some women also viewed couples' testing in positive terms. Mildred, a 30-year-old mother of five, told me that having an HIV-negative outcome as a couple could reinforce prevention strategies for the remainder of the pregnancy: "It helps because … if you find that you are still fine then the two of you should stay well in the house." I asked Mildred to elaborate on what she meant by "staying well," and she explained:

> Keeping oneself well is, when you have both tested and found that you are both healthy, as a woman you should not get many men. The man should not also get many women. You should stay the way you have tested because there isn't anything bad in your body, so you should keep those children you are producing.

Mildred also believed that the negative test was a sign that her husband had been faithful to her and her co-wife: "At the time we began staying with my co [-wife], we went and tested and found that up to now, he has not yet added anybody on to the two of us." Learning their negative status reassured her about the well-being of herself and her unborn baby and the faithfulness within her polygamous marriage. Polygynous marriages are commonplace in this area (Westerhaus et al., 2007; Patel et al., 2014a) including among study participants. Like Mildred, Kelly found the test reassuring because she doubted her husband's fidelity: "When I was pregnant and it had just begun, I thought that I was HIV positive, a disease that people fear so much. We had tested and had found out that we were not HIV positive, but fear only existed because my husband is not very morally upright." The link between men's infidelity and the likelihood of contracting HIV made testing a situation in which marriages were under scrutiny in a way that was not always comfortable, particularly for the unfaithful partner. This discomfort contributed to male reluctance to test.

The potential for blame or violence was part of the context through which participants assessed couples' testing. Some participants saw couples' testing as ameliorating negative impacts of disclosure. For example, Leah told me: "It is good, because if you went alone he would change to say he was healthy so you are the one who brought the sickness." Annette, a focus group participant in Pagak, offered the following stark assessment:

> Another benefit of going to hospital with the man is that when you find you are positive you can be counselled together, and it is helpful, because if the woman finds she is positive it becomes difficult to tell the man. That's why we hardly tell them. That is why the medics tell us to go together – so that after, we may get support and live positively. You may come back and tell him your status and he cuts you with a *panga* [machete] and you die. So it is better to know together – he could have actually even have brought the sickness.

Her hypothetical example demonstrates how fear of violent reprisal for a positive HIV status made HIV testing and disclosure a risky prospect for women.

While concern over violence resulting from blame is one rationale for testing and counselling to occur for both partners simultaneously, it was clear from speaking to women that the couples' test had not resolved the problem of violence. Fear of violence could also shape women's ability to recruit their husbands to attend care. In a study in eastern Uganda, women also recounted feeling compelled to negotiate their husbands' participation: "The majority described it as a complicated mission and a major dilemma to try to recruit their spouses while having very limited power to influence their partner's actions" (Larsson et al., 2012, p. 4). The anxiety associated with recruiting partners was attached to the fear of male violence. While voluntary couples' testing can avoid the blame and violence these women describe, compulsory couples' testing initiated by the women's health care providers reinforced gendered power relations. In Amuru, women were held responsible for persuading men to test and were then required to live through the consequences associated with positive status and disclosure, as well as with male refusal to attend.

## Health Worker Perspectives on Couples' HIV Testing During ANC

Health workers attributed men's reluctance to test for HIV in part to factors similar to those described by the mothers, including men's tendency to see pregnancy as a "woman's problem" and their fear of a positive test. Along with these shared themes, health workers identified the health centre environment, gender norms among their patients, and logistical factors as contributing to men's low participation. To counter male reluctance, health workers employed various methods. These included providing incentives for men to attend, creating barriers to women whose husbands refused to attend, and introducing punishments for men who refused to attend. These strategies had negative repercussions for pregnant women's relationships and health care.

I asked health workers for their thoughts on why men were reluctant to test. Dorothy, a nurse aide, said that the difficulty of transportation and male perceptions that pregnancy was solely a woman's concern contributed to the challenges women had in persuading male partners to attend. She explained:

> Say you tell them [husbands] about antenatal care, some of them may refuse. So some say there's no transport, others they say it's not their problem. (Sarah): It's not their problem. (Dorothy): Yeah, because they are not the one who is pregnant.

When I asked Amy, a nursing assistant, about men who refuse to attend, she shared two possibilities: men's knowledge of a positive status that they did not want to disclose, or men's belief that their wife's test would suffice for both partners. She explained:

> Maybe that husband, you know with men, they are so perseverant, unh? Maybe he had known before that woman is coming to the hospital [health

centre] for medical check-up, maybe he had known already that he was
already positive (Sarah): mm (Amy): and he will not allow, or not involve
himself to the hospital just simply because, they will feel ashamed, now, they
are going to pinpoint me that "have you seen that man, that man is already
positive."

Here, Amy is referring to the stigma that is still very much attached to
HIV. She also cited men's refrain as "If you are positive, it means I am
positive. And if you are negative, I am negative. Because we are one."
She emphasized to me that "they always tell it like that, you see?" Overall, Amy was frustrated with men's approach to testing. She said, "If I am
to tell it they are so negligent, eh, they are negligent … They want to
neglect their what? Their wives." While she understood that men felt
shame or might perceive one test among the couple to be sufficient, she
also regarded men who refused to attend in negative terms. I found her
frustration with a perceived negligence or neglect to be understandable
yet recognized that such perceptions have the potential to detract from
efforts to address men's fears and misconceptions about HIV and testing.
Rather than restricting blame to men or to gender relations within the
local culture, the role of policies and practices needs to be adequately
scrutinized.

Logistical and social factors intersected to create the conditions for
male resistance to HIV testing. Lack of privacy at the health centre and
the pressures of childcare and farm work at home made it difficult for
both partners to be away simultaneously. The DHO, Peter, felt that the
health centre environment reinforced men's negative perceptions of
participation:

The environment in the health centre is not attractive for men. You are
going into one room which is full of women only, a man sitting there would
definitely feel out of place, is one. Then from the cultural point of view, a
man who is seen moving with the wife, moving in the antenatal, and accompanying the wife everywhere, there is belief in the culture that this man has
been overpowered by the woman.

Just as Peter described, on a typical day the health centre was a predominantly female space: a majority of patients were children accompanied
by women, while the staff was mostly made up of women, with men tend-
ing to fill higher-status positions and therefore being less visible, working in private offices or in the lab. The fear of emasculation and other
gendered norms of behaviour were influential in governing men's view
that their role in pregnancy should be limited, Peter argued, and this

was exacerbated by the unsuitability of the health centre environment. Betty, a focus group participant in Pagak, similarly suggested changes to the waiting area; men and women should be instructed to stay together, and a toilet and drinking water station should be attached to the waiting area. She felt this would solve a problem with men leaving during testing, either while waiting for the test or for results. With such changes, men could not pretend to step out for a drink or to use the bathroom. As Peter saw it, the interplay between gendered expectations and inadequate facilities contributed to male reluctance to attend ANC and test for HIV.

Other challenges to male ANC attendance and couples' testing arose from the context of poverty, poor infrastructure, and subsistence agriculture. Peter shared the following:

> Then there are the economic and social issues. Instead of transporting the mother alone, you may need two people. The cost involved, the issue of distance … Then, you see, if they are very far away, the mother can go some days before the antenatal care, say from deep in the village. She can stay with a relative around the health center. They see you in the clinic you can stay there and go back … But then you cannot bring a whole couple. At least one person has to stay back to look after the children, the property, and things like that.

As discussed in chapter 3, transportation costs and challenges were substantial. Larger family sizes and the reliance on agriculture meant that concerns about managing the work at home were considerable, particularly for remote families where an ANC visit might necessitate an overnight absence. These responsibilities affected the extent to which couples' could attend ANC together. As I worked to understand the influence of various dynamic factors, it became clear to me how social relations and health care approaches shape each other; gender norms are not static but are shaped by external factors.

## Health Worker Strategies for Couples' Testing in the Face of Male Reluctance

Despite the male reluctance described, health workers were tasked with ensuring as many men as possible were tested in order to meet their goals around preventing vertical transmission of HIV. Strategies to promote male attendance at the first ANC appointment and HIV testing included health education, the requirement for women to bring an LC I letter stating that their husband was dead or unable to participate, and positive reinforcement for husbands who did participate. The LC I letter functioned as a text that coordinated pregnant women's activities and those of their partners with the goals of the health centre and, beyond that, national and international goals on HIV prevention. Requiring the LC I letter also changed the role of health providers in relation to their patients, introducing an administrative, ruling relation function; it required health workers not only to care for the patient in front of them but also to intervene to persuade them to bring their husbands. Local strategies were reportedly effective in increasing male participation yet had negative consequences for some women's lives.

The LC I letter was a particular hurdle for women whose partners refused to attend ANC. In collaboration with the local political leaders (the LC), health workers insisted that women whose husbands would not participate or were absent get a letter written by an LC I. This meant women had to visit a political leader to plead their case. The paternalism of such an approach is undeniable, but what worried me more was how this requirement created additional work for a woman in arranging her ANC care and had the potential to delay care or act as a barrier to receiving care. LC I letters did not typically state that the husband had refused to attend; instead, the letters made the assertion that the husband was dead or in prison. The assumption was that there was, in fact, an involved male partner who acknowledged paternity and was in a marriage-like partnership with the mother. However, of course, this was not always the case. The protocol of the LC I letter stigmatized single women. Acero, my RA, believed women would prefer not to share their single status, telling me "you don't pierce your own eye" (similar to the admonition against airing one's dirty laundry). Creating additional negative consequences for single mothers exacerbated the stigma and exceptionalism directed at them. The way husbands were brought into ANC reaffirmed Christian, patriarchal family norms by reiterating a two-parent heterosexual family as normative, part of a larger social context of extreme heteronormativity. It further marginalized women who were alone due to unwanted pregnancies, family breakdown, or an absent partner. While norms around marriage and family are most commonly described as cultural and localized in nature, such norms can be informed by and policed by health care policies and practices. The requirement of the involvement of local leaders in the case of men who were reluctant to attend ANC and test for HIV policed women whose families did not fit a rigid norm or whose husbands refused to comply. At the same time, it reinforced the sense that this participation was compulsory rather than voluntary.

The midwife Gloria described how an LC I letter was an additional step to take, if necessary, after educating communities to understand that men should attend the first ANC appointment:

So pertaining to the men, in order to come with their women to antenatal care, ... first of all we just health-educate them generally, about the goodness of attending antenatal with their partners together ... secondly, if a mother comes without the partner, we, at least me, we inquire her to get the letters from the LC ... On that she will find is very difficult, and then she will go back to the husband and say "let's go to the hospital" and then they will come.

She and Grace, the other midwife, saw the approach of requiring an LC I letter as effective, as demonstrated by the following exchange between the two midwives and me:

(Grace): It's hard to make them come, but we still tell them you have to come. If you cannot come, bring for us the letter from the LC. If today I go to the LC, my husband refuse, tomorrow, do you think again I will go? It's hard. So by that, few would go. (Sarah): Okay. (Gloria): Very few, those ones who don't have really the husband around which at least go. So that is the only way we could make them at least try their best. So there are some few who come without. (Grace): Most of them come with their partners. (Gloria): Currently very few come without. Of ten people, only two or one.

In identifying the difficulty of getting an LC I letter, Grace made it clear that the requirement was a way of exerting pressure on women to facilitate male involvement. As well as creating the impression that couples' testing was mandatory, the letter acted as a deliberate hurdle to health care for women whose husbands wanted to opt out. An innovation created to meet the demands of the MDGs, the LC letter was an example of how an international policy that did not specify coercion nevertheless resulted in coercive practices. Caught up in these ruling relations, the midwives worked to implement the LC I letter, evidently not recognizing the work that this created for their patients or the tension it created between the primary care function of their work and the policing role they were asked to take on.

Another strategy used by one village leader (LC I) was to require men who refused to test to do community service, usually slashing the tall grass surrounding a village compound or path. An LC I who required this told me that at a group meeting of leaders there had been discussion of implementing this strategy throughout the sub-county. Coercive strategies to promote changes in health-related behaviour were not unique to maternity care; this type of punishment was also extended to people who refused to have their homes sprayed with insecticide to prevent malaria. However, such strategies disproportionately impacted pregnant women because of local politics, gendered relations, and women's dependence on health care workers for care.

The nursing assistant, Amy, explained to me some of the tactics that she used to increase attendance on the part of men. She felt that presenting an LC I letter was not sufficient, since the letter would state the husband was dead or in prison when it was more typically the case that he was simply refusing to attend. She said:

> And when they say the husband has died, we are going to prove. (Sarah): Okay? (Amy): We prove it in this way: that when did your husband die? They may tell you that "oh my husband, my husband died last year in November." For example now we are in August, eh? We prove it like that, that where did you get this pregnancy … And then, if we take it short like that, short-cut, eh they start to tell us the truth. That, "Unh-unh, no nurse, my husband refused to come to the hospital." (Sarah): Okay. (Amy): They tell you the fact. And that is how we even grab them so they come in. (Sarah): And then you get the husbands. (Amy): We say when you go back home, tell your husband for the next time you come. Some will come, some will still deny. They will tell you that "unh-unh, nurse, the husband refuses totally."

Amy used the LC I letter as an opportunity to get the "truth" about a husband's whereabouts. As her example demonstrates, women experienced facilitating their husbands' participation similarly to participants elsewhere in Uganda as a "complicated mission and a major dilemma" (Larsson et al., 2012, p. 4).

Amy also told me how incentives could be used to encourage male antenatal participation. She said that the mama kits were a form of encouragement for men as well as women: "Now that thing has encouraged those husbands and the wives, to encourage themselves to come to hospital [the health centre]." She described an example in which the soap from the kits had been provided to men who attended ANC, leading to an increase in male attendance. She went on to say,

> And that is one side, we always motivate them. When you find something that is providable to them, you always give it to them so that they encourage them to visit health centre regularly.

This strategy, while seen by health workers as an effective form of motivation, complemented the practice of punishing men who refused to attend. Both were measures to manipulate men into participating in ANC and testing. It also contributed to the scarcity of Red Cross project supplies since there was a limited amount of soap for the mama kits.

However, neither practice directly addressed the social and logistical barriers to male participation. These reasons, including inequitable gender relations, the practical difficulty of both adults simultaneously leaving the work of home, and logistical factors at the health centre, were important but overlooked.

While requiring the LC I letter was coercive, health workers saw such strategies as effective and positive because of a visible increase in the numbers of men participating in couples' testing, which indicated that a goal was being met. However, in their focus on the numbers, a focus encouraged by the demand for metrics in international approaches to maternal health and HIV transmission, health workers appeared to have overlooked the work and difficulties created in the lives of their patients. A focus on metrics was evident in Jonas's assertion that filling in monitoring forms well enough to "satisfy someone" was a weakness among junior staff. Their approach created work for women whose husbands were initially reluctant as it fell to them to come up with persuasion strategies. For others, it was the work involved in obtaining an LC I letter. Beyond the time, effort, and strategizing of work, women risked facing other serious repercussions. These included male drunkenness and violence, evidenced by the participant who worried over the possibility of being attacked with a machete.

A gap between valuing the numbers of people tested for HIV and valuing women's rights and access to health care more broadly was also identified by Angotti et al. (2011), who argue that while coercive approaches to routine testing did result in an increase in those tested, this happened at the expense of "the individual rights of pregnant women" (p. 34). They conclude that "the social relations in which HIV testing occurs in rural Malawi may not represent the idealized notions assumed by global or national policies" (p. 314). Going beyond this, I suggest not only that existing social relations are more complex than the neutral or idealized picture assumed by policy approaches, but that policy approaches themselves can actively shape social relations in problematic ways. In Amuru, when the broader picture of rights, social relations, and access to care is considered, the current policy and practice approach to HIV testing during ANC falls short. Understanding these shortcomings contributes to working towards equitable access to care.

### "Without a Man We Are Not Going to Give You a Card": Male Refusal as a Barrier to Women's Care

Compulsory approaches to couples' HIV testing during ANC discouraged or impeded care for some pregnant or birthing women. Being refused care was something the women who I interviewed worried about, talked about, and planned their approach to maternity care and childbirth around. Women might opt out of ANC and health centre delivery if they believed they were going to be turned away. Meanwhile, health workers used this fear of being refused care as a strategy to increase male partner participation.

In our conversation, Jonas was aware of the relationship between male reluctance and whether women attended a full complement of ANC:

> Men still do not focus much on the health of women during pregnancy … When these women get pregnant we want them to come for antenatal with their husbands but some husbands they do not turn up during the antenatal so you find that the woman will fear to come also alone and attend the antenatal clinic and this makes most women to come very late for antenatal care. As a result, you find that some attend only once or twice during the pregnancy, which is actually not what is expected.

Jonas had concluded that when men were expected to participate in ANC and did not want to, women's participation was detrimentally affected. Within focused ANC, the number of visits is already small in comparison to ANC provision in the global north, as described in chapter 3. Ideally, the health system would be working to facilitate ANC visits in the face of transportation and other difficulties; introducing a hindrance to care is a major misstep. Missing visits meant that opportunities to identify or treat complications or otherwise meet women's needs were lost, putting maternal-child health at risk.

If it was difficult for women to attend ANC because of male partner reluctance, those who wanted a facility-based delivery had to persevere, since ANC was structured as a gateway to delivery care. Although health centre staff maintained that women without an ANC card would not be turned away at the time of labour, an ANC card was nevertheless perceived by childbearing women and described by health staff as necessary to receive delivery care at a health centre. It gradually became clear to me that beyond documenting basic health information – its function on the face of things – the ANC card had become an important text coordinating access to care. Gloria, a midwife, was aware that women who wanted to give birth at the health centre were unlikely to opt out of ANC and would do their best to comply. When I asked, "Do you think women ever avoid antenatal care because of this policy [couples' testing], or not?" she replied:

> They can't avoid, because they know that when they come in labour, or in case of any problem, they need antenatal care, they have to have the card.

> All of them in the village know that without antenatal care it is not easy to go for delivery when they are in labour.

Gloria's conception of the role of the ANC card echoed that of the women cited in chapter 4, who saw the card as a ticket to giving birth in the health centre. This strategy was coercive; care during labour should be an entitlement, not a benefit that women have to earn. Further, rather than emphasizing ANC care, couples' HIV testing, and delivery care as interlocking aspects of health care for pregnant women, this strategy made each stage of care contingent on the prior stage. For women experiencing a barrier to couples' testing, this barrier was reproduced at later ANC appointments and particularly at the time of delivery.

The health workers I interviewed perceived couples' testing during ANC as beneficial to women. For example, Gloria identified HIV testing as one of two main reasons ANC was important to her clients, when asked to speculate as to what patients valued in ANC. (The second reason was to learn of any complications of pregnancy that would require a hospital trip so women could save for transport accordingly.) Gloria described the value of testing as follows: "At least they know their status. Some may go two years without testing, but when you are pregnant, you must. At least they know their status and the advice. If they are positive, they are advised the way of life." HIV testing was beneficial to women themselves, beyond its role in PMTCT; perhaps this benefit contributed to health worker's willingness to police male testing.

Participants saw male involvement in ANC as facilitating their future care. A focus group participant, Betty, said that without men's cooperation, women might miss essential care:

> Another benefit of going to hospital with the man is that once you are tested, you, the woman, are given some medicine that is said to help even the baby. So the pain is, when the man runs away and you miss it. Like the vitamins, because they give like three types of drugs which you swallow, and it is not good to miss all when the men run away.

Betty may have been referring to folic acid, iron, and a malaria prophylaxis, all offered as part of ANC. Her comment was based on the perception that couples' testing was mandatory and that without it, health care such as medication might be denied. When HIV testing, ANC, and health centre delivery were each seen as compulsory, childbearing women believed each stage of care to be contingent on their compliance with previous stages. These findings echo those of Larsson et al.'s (2012) study, which suggested that "if testing is perceived as compulsory it could potentially deter some women from seeking ANC services" (p. 6). As the participant quoted above observed, missing part of ANC has negative consequences for the health of women and their babies.

The midwife Gloria shared some background on the approach to couples' testing that suggested that making future care contingent on male participation had been a deliberate strategy. Asked when the health centre had started to implement couples' testing during ANC, she told me, "It was since before, but no one really put a male focus on it. Until when we said '*without a man we are not going to give you a card.*' They will try now" (my italics). Treating the male partner as a gateway to ANC reproduces gendered power imbalances in relationships, as well as barriers in accessing ANC – complicating the structural context shaping women's experiences of and access to maternity care. Dorothy, a nurse aide, told me that "if the husband has refused to accompany the mother, we do take the blood of the mother, but ask them for the second time when they come, they need to come up with the husband." However, Amelia, a participant, told me that "when you have reached [the health centre] for ANC without your husband, the health worker doesn't test you [for HIV]." Women, she said, were made to wait until they could be present with a husband who was also willing to be tested. Betty said, "They give cards but without results, each time you went they would remind you to go together to receive your results. They actually scare you that you won't deliver at hospital if you didn't come for results." Penny, a 29-year-old mother who had lost her firstborn and had five living children, explained to me that she could not persuade her husband to attend ANC or to test for HIV during her most recent pregnancy, so she continued care without him. After her first visit, she recounted:

> So when I went back alone they didn't disturb me until I completed my ANC. They tested and it was negative, and though they also wanted my husband's results, he did not ever reach there until my due date reached and I delivered without him testing.

Penny indirectly attributed her husband's absence from ANC to infidelity and to alcohol use, telling me that "men sometimes don't like to be tested. I think because of the alcohol they take. Sometimes they mess around." Overall, the threat that without male participation, access to care would be denied to women was used as a way of coercing women to mobilize men. This coercive measure affected access to care and the relationships between childbearing women and their care providers.

Access to ANC was already challenging for women; it was curtailed by poverty, transportation difficulties, and lack of resources, among other issues. The importance of PMTCT notwithstanding, encouraging male participation in ANC and HIV testing should not have come at the expense of birthing women's participation in ANC and facility-based delivery.

Because TBAs were discouraged from attending births, and were not formally part of ANC, they did not feature in the strategy on couples' testing except insofar as they were told to refer pregnant women and their partners to the health centre. Nevertheless, TBAs of course worried over HIV status and the risks they faced. After holding two focus groups with TBAs, I wrote in my field notes:

> Even here, HIV is really playing into things. First, it seems to me that the TBAs have been told that avoiding HIV is a major reason that their assistance with homebirths is so discouraged. And then, they are still sometimes at deliveries. Yet, they can't, and desperately want to be able to, understand whether a woman's ANC card says she is HIV positive or not. They want to use this, and then be able to tactfully say, "oh, your situation is complicated, you should go to the health centre." Also, they want gloves. I am wondering whether not offering such training, and not supplying with gloves … is part of the strategy to prevent the work of TBAs delivering in the village. If so, then, the unfortunate consequence might be around HIV prevention (as they end up delivering but without these two tools that might help with prevention).

This tension also speaks to the failure to truly integrate an HIV-prevention strategy with a skilled birth strategy.

### Gender, Couples' Testing, and Vertical Health

While male involvement is important for PMTCT and can support the health of both partners, I learned that implementing couples' testing is not straightforward. The pressures on relationships arising from testing can be serious, potentially leading to violence and the dissolution of relationships. Women who test without their partners and are positive can face severe consequences including "blame and abandonment" (Medley et al., 2012, p. 361). While testing together is looked to as a means of reducing the potential for blame, stigma attached to the disease can fuel men's reluctance to be tested. For such reasons, identifying HIV during pregnancy for the purposes of PMTCT is a challenge for health systems in many sub-Saharan African countries. It is not unusual for health facilities to resort to coercion (Hardon et al., 2012), such as was the case for women testing in Malawi (Angotti et al., 2011) as well as elsewhere in Uganda. A study set in eastern Uganda found that "HIV testing was viewed as compulsory" and made the case that this affirmed "recent concerns that the global policy change from VCT [voluntary counselling and testing] to provider-initiated HIV testing could make patients feel obliged to test" (Larsson et al., 2012 p. 5). As in Amuru, "very few men spontaneously accompanied their wives for ANC, health workers tried to recruit men for testing through the pregnant women" (p. 5), and the absence of male partners was viewed as the responsibility of women (p. 2). Coercive practices have gained authority in Uganda via the recently passed the *HIV and AIDS Prevention and Control Act, 2014* (Republic of Uganda, 2014; see also Devi, 2014). This Act criminalizes HIV transmission, allows health workers to disclose patients' status in certain circumstances, and makes HIV testing mandatory for women and their partners, a change since the research was undertaken. As laws criminalizing HIV transmission are replicated in sub-Saharan African countries (Grace, 2015), it is likely that more countries will make HIV testing compulsory for pregnant women and their intimate partners. Already, testing is heavily regulated and transmission increasingly criminalized in several sub-Saharan African countries, especially in west Africa: "Guinea's HIV law makes HIV tests mandatory before marriage; and Sierra Leone's HIV law explicitly criminalizes a mother living with HIV who exposes her child or fetus to HIV" (Pearshouse, 2014, p. 14). The stakes for understanding how compulsory testing affects access to care and violence in intimate relationships are therefore high.

One major feature of global health recommendations that did not get taken up in practice in Amuru was the voluntary and coercion-free approach specified by global health organizations including the WHO. Specifically, the WHO and UNAIDS (the Joint United Nations Program on HIV/AIDS) guidelines for provider-initiated HIV testing state:

> Patients must receive adequate information on which to base a personal and voluntary decision whether or not to consent to the test, and be given an explicit opportunity to decline a recommendation of HIV testing and counselling without coercion. (WHO, 2007, p. 33, as cited in Angotti et al., 2011, p. 308)

This disjuncture between a model described as voluntary and a local implementation and perception of testing as compulsory has been identified elsewhere in sub-Saharan Africa. In Malawi, researchers examined perceptions of HIV testing during pregnancy and found that "rural Malawians do not perceive HIV testing as a choice, but rather as compulsory in order to receive antenatal care" (Angotti et al., 2011, p. 307).

This perception arose despite a national policy identifying that "women must be explicitly informed of their right to refuse testing," (p. 307) an approach backed by international policy. The study, which focused on women's testing (not couples' testing), concluded that there is a "dissonance between global expectations and local realities of the delivery of HIV-testing interventions" (Angotti et al., 2011, p. 307). Such dissonance had an impact on women's personal relationships and their approaches to antenatal and delivery care. As in the Malawi case, participants in Amuru perceived couple' testing during ANC to be "an offer you can't refuse."

Health worker participants described implementing couples' testing during ANC as part of a national policy that responded to international goals. The DHO, Peter, characterized couples' testing during ANC as such. When I asked, "And so the HIV testing of husbands at ANC and the requirement for men to attend, that's district-wide, or nation-wide?" Peter responded by saying, "It's a national policy, a Ministry of Health policy they have come up with." The testing practices at the health centre were shaped by the national policy context and by the international policy context, including the MDGs, despite reflecting these policy contexts imperfectly. Midwife Gloria also pointed out this connection between HIV testing practices at the health centre and a national program that, in turn, responded to the MDGs to be achieved by 2015. She stated in an interview:

> Pertaining to men coming to antenatal care, that one is based on the government program where by 2015 no babies will be born with HIV infection. (Sarah): Right. (Gloria): Now in that, they are suggesting, they feel if they can make all males, it is a routine and it is a must for all males to be tested. Because I can be negative and my husband can be positive. I can get it anytime during pregnancy.

These national and local approaches, then, responded to global approaches and goals, including the MDGs. However, in this case, some of the features that were discarded in implementation were those crucial to women's rights and safety.

In identifying couples' testing as a national policy and an iteration of global health policies, Peter also described problems in its implementation that emerged as gender relations:

> But the challenge is how to get the men in the health facility. He is not going to come. There was a time they tried to put it as a regulation that any mother who comes with a husband is attended to first. What they discovered later on was that it was no longer the wives bringing their husband, but

> they were bringing any male. So we find if a mother is coming for antenatal, there is a *boda-boda* transporting her … [laughter] That [the motorcycle-taxi driver] would be the husband. So the whole policy lost meaning.

The tactic of using men as proxy husbands revealed the women's strong desire to receive ANC but also signalled that powerful norms and ideals influencing men's actions and inactions also affected women's access to ANC and delivery care. Rewarding women who brought their husbands to ANC was a failed attempt at regulation since women's "compliance" took the form of being accompanied by *any* man, not necessarily their husband, in an unintended consequence of the policy. The difficulty of mobilizing male partner involvement, then, was a challenge for policymakers, as well as for health workers and birthing women. While gender dynamics such as men's refusal to test are often attributed to cultural contexts, it is important to recognize that health policies can also exert pressure on social relations, at times amplifying rather than diminishing gendered inequities.

One problem with the policy approach is that maternal health and HIV prevention were approached separately, as though they were unrelated. This allowed for the approach to HIV testing, which supported MDG 6 (to combat HIV) to be carried out in such a way that it undermined access to ANC, critical to MDG 5 (to improve maternal health). This is a persistent structural problem that occurs because of a preference for vertical health approaches. Vertical health addresses global health challenges via disease- or intervention-specific silos, in contrast to horizontal health interventions, which emphasize cross-cutting supports to health, typically via investments in health systems or health care personnel. A vertical approach to health interventions creates competition for funding and recognition among initiatives (Filippi et al., 2006). The vertical approach is often observed to be "donor-driven and technocratic" (Magnussen et al., 2004, p. 169). An emphasis on vertical programs comes at the expense of "emphasis on development and sustainability of health systems and infrastructures" (Magnussen et al., 2004, p. 169). This occurs in spite of the Declaration of Alma Ata (1978), which identified primary health care as the best means of working towards "health for all," a principle subsequently adopted by the WHO. The need to shift course was recognized in a 2018 *Lancet* editorial, in which Pamela Das and Richard Horton argue that "it is now time to end the siloed and vertical response to AIDS" (p. 260). Dickinson et al. (2009) observe that although linkages between reproductive and sexual health and HIV programming are "feasible and beneficial," they are rarely implemented. Within Uganda, the integration of HIV and ANC has, in fact, been piloted. However, a qualitative study tracing the pilot integration in two districts found major challenges to integration stemming, primarily, from lack of health system capacity on various fronts (Ahumuza et al., 2016). In the case of Amuru, an approach to HIV prevention that also supported other aspects of maternity health care was necessary to avoid the access problems created when women's future care depended on male compliance with the couples' test.

## Gender and Intersectional Power Relationships

The clinical officer in-charge, Jonas, identified the twofold purpose of having male partners attend the first ANC appointment. First, he emphasized, was the prevention of mother-to-child transmission of HIV (PMTCT) and planning for care according to HIV status. He went on to say, "The second part is, okay, men are being encouraged to get more close, and take more responsibility to their pregnant women." While my analysis focuses on practices surrounding the goal of PMTCT through testing, the second goal – raising men's awareness of and value for women's health during pregnancy – demonstrates how health policies can have effects beyond the clinical and shape social relations both intentionally and unintentionally. Health providers worked to be a part of men's shifting gender roles in relation to maternity care and birth; however, much of this took place via men's female partners or via responsibilization messaging that failed to account for factors structuring men's reluctance. Gender relations are a major feature of the social context of HIV prevention, testing, and disclosure within the context of pregnancy and birth. Efforts at HIV prevention need to intersect with efforts to counter gendered violence. Targeting men via women compromises such a goal.

When discussing the difficulties participants face in bringing their husbands to ANC, it is necessary to recognize that gender norms within Acholi culture are neither monolithic nor static. Participants shared stories of husbands whose involvement was difficult or impossible to negotiate, as well as of husbands who approached pregnancy and parenting with support. Husbands' support was evident, for example, in efforts to save money for supplies for the birth and the new child. As well, some participants' husbands willingly agreed to participate in the first appointment and to test for HIV, for their own sake and that of their families. For example, Monica, who had a constantly nursing one-year-old and said she was now expecting her ninth child, told us that her husband "thinks of his health."

While the reluctance of some men to test can be regarded as irresponsible by their partners and by health workers, another way of understanding it is to recognize that HIV was feared within the community (as elsewhere) and that learning of a positive status was life-changing. Furthermore, couples' HIV testing occurred within a context that could be difficult for men. Participants linked men's overuse of alcohol to their tendency to have extramarital sex and to avoid testing. Alcohol dependency must be understood, in part, as a response to traumas survived during the conflict period, as well as the subsequent economic and social impacts on day-to-day life, and it is linked to intimate partner violence (Annan & Brier, 2010). Many of the men whom women spoke about were likely to be survivors of, or witnesses to, atrocious violence. Examining the links between the conflict and displacement and how masculinity is expressed, Oosterom (2011) writes that during the protracted conflict,

> unable to meet societal expectations, men became frustrated, which was described by some as prompting feelings of humiliation. This caused various social and psychological problems, such as alcoholism, suicide attempts, and engaging in violence in fights or domestic violence and also caused some men to join the armed forces. It could also lead to the perpetration of psychological violence, through the suppression of the less powerful, such as women and youth. This has affected women's position in Acholi society. (p. 400)

Shifting gender roles affected work and power in intimate relationships in ways that made life more difficult for women. Oosterom (2011) found that in the camps, women's responsibilities increased as they undertook work previously done by men. These changes, she argues, have become entrenched in the post-conflict period (p. 404). Others also noted an increase in women's responsibilities: "With the semi-urban lifestyles that evolved in camps and the impact of globalisation, there are changes to gender roles, with women taking on more responsibilities that used to be exclusively male dominated and the tensions that may arise from this" (Omona & Aduo, 2013, p. 132). War was also a contributor to male violence against women, as "the rate of domestic violence increased seriously during the insurgency, and many women still face violence to their bodies on a daily basis. One woman stated succinctly: 'As long as there is no peace in our homes, the war is not over'" (Oosterom, 2011, p. 404). Such concerns contribute to the everyday social context within which women coordinate their maternity care and birth.

Approaches to health care must consider gender relations within the historical and intergenerational effects of conflict. Westerhaus et al. (2007) describe the connection between displacement and violence, and make the case that "HIV prevention programs must acknowledge these realities and attempt to counter this violence by working with men to reshape their gender roles in ways that are acceptable to both men and women" (p. 1185). Larsson et al. (2012) share the concern that similar approaches to testing fail to integrate the inseparable connection between gender and power. They assert that despite WHO emphasis on integrating gender into health policy, "gender aspects in terms of decision-making power and women's financial dependency on their male partners is rarely integrated in policy development and implementation" (p. 6). Gender-sensitive implementation, they suggest, might target men directly, such as through peer-education or clinics, instead of through their pregnant wives.

Just as a partner's support is crucial for women during pregnancy and around birth, the consequences of an unsupportive, difficult, or violent marriage can be amplified during this time. Male reluctance to test can only be partially understood in terms of gender relations within marriage; it is also shaped by forces such as health care practices, politics, and priorities.

## Conclusion

Approaches to HIV surveillance, access to ANC, and men's perceived social roles in their partner's pregnancy acted as a structural context within which maternity care and birth were socially organized in Amuru. Voluntary, provider-initiated couples' testing, presented and perceived as mandatory, had negative impacts on women who were pregnant, notwithstanding its positive contribution to PMTCT. Coupled with male reluctance shaped by gender norms, patriarchal power relations, and logistical factors, the compulsory approach to testing resulted in additional work for women, contributed to the potential for blame and violence, and curtailed access to care, all of which could adversely influence pregnancy and birth outcomes. While women were exhorted to seek formal care provision during pregnancy, the ways in which care was offered at times presented disincentives and barriers to their participation. A discourse of empowerment and choice is a poor fit within this context; as MacKian (2008) writes, "Although the current policy climate aims to encourage women to utilise formal health provision, they are often the least able to negotiate access effectively" (p. 112). The gendered and intersectional dimensions of power at play in current approaches to HIV testing point to a need for better policy options. Both the failures of coercion and the perceived need for such an approach demonstrate the necessity for a more direct approach in targeting men and, more broadly, in facilitating optimal approaches to HIV prevention within the context of pregnancy. The approach to HIV testing during ANC in Amuru sub-county acknowledges the importance of men's role and participation, yet simultaneously reproduces existing gender and social inequities. The potential for public health interventions to amplify rather than diminish inequalities is documented in various contexts (Fleming et al., 2014; Thompson & Kumar, 2011); this is particularly crucial in reproductive and sexual health, where gender relations are so strongly at play.

# Chapter Six

# Conclusions: Reconceiving the Maternal Health Crisis

## Introduction

At the outset of this book, I described a legal struggle to recognize the deaths of two women in childbirth as the Ugandan government's failure to provide care. The allegations were underpinned by the claim that a lack of basic supplies, including sutures, had compromised care and led to the untimely and unnecessary deaths of women in state health care facilities. This is an example of "landmark litigation ... establishing important precedents regarding the obligation of government to provide reproductive health care" (Yamin, 2013, p. 2). The case succeeded, and this obligation is now part of public discourse.

On a 2019 visit, while driving to the capital, I saw a roadside billboard proclaiming that "citizens have a right to proper health care" (see Figure 6.1). This was a project of the Uganda Debt Network, which lobbies on poverty-related issues, and centred the financial aspect of the crisis in care. It displayed a cartoon narrative showing how corruption at government-run facilities has created the need for citizens to purchase their own medications and supplies, ultimately leading to unnecessary deaths. The billboard depicted failed health care for a pregnant woman, the final panel portraying her burial with the husband lamenting, "Now my wife is dead."

The strategic litigation and the public message centring health rights signal a refusal to accept maternal mortality as inevitable. They call to mind observations made by Farmer (2008), who, witnessing the poor conditions in a Malawi maternity ward, attributed the country's shocking maternal mortality rate of 18,000/100,000 to intersecting oppressions constituted by gender inequity and poverty. He argued that the reduction of maternal mortality is a human rights issue that depends on access to quality care, asking, "Should there be a right to sutures? To sterile

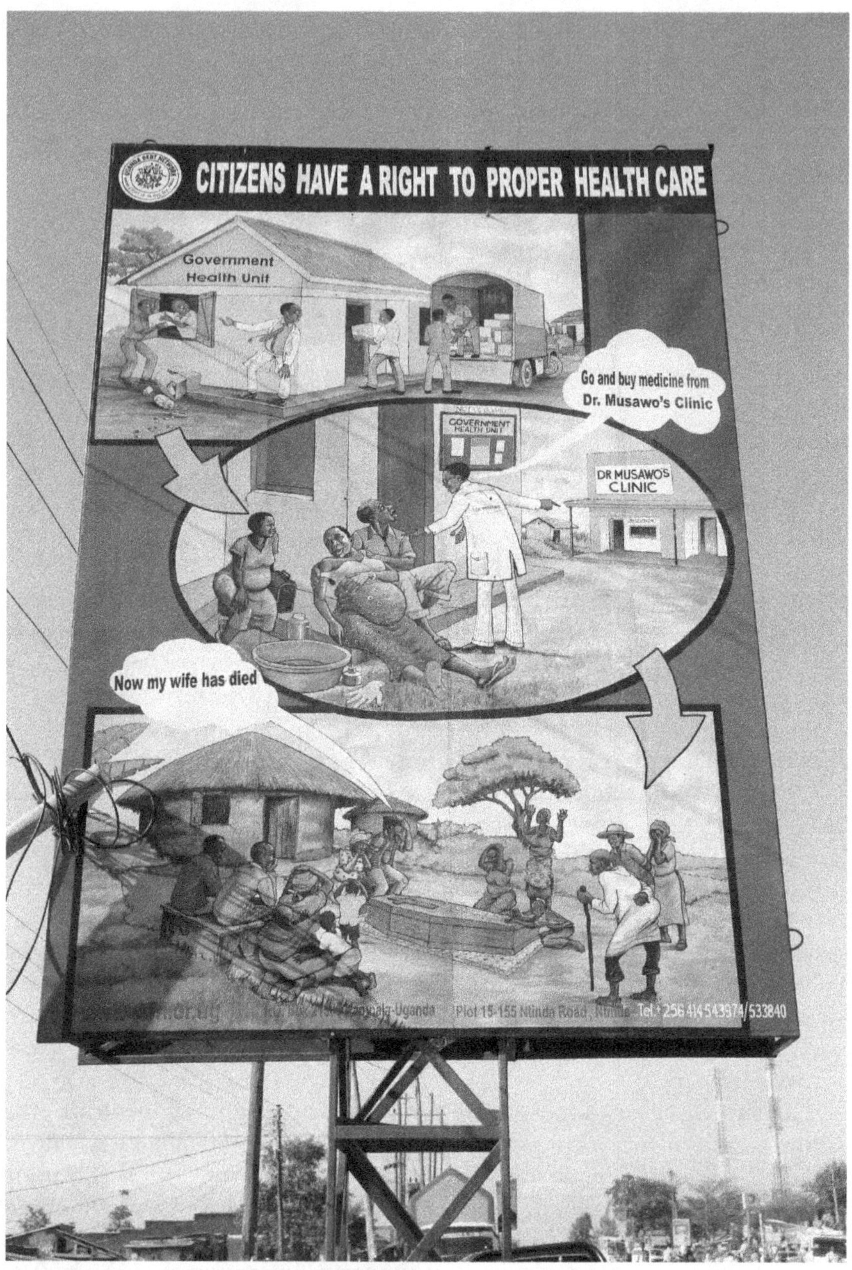


Figure 6.1.  Citizens have a right to proper health care. Roadside sign between Gulu and Kampala. (Source: Godong/Alamy Stock Photo.)

drapes? To anesthesia?" (p. 4). Social justice, access to basic maternity supplies, and the provision of care in clinical settings are interrelated forces shaping maternity health care and maternal mortality (Venkatapuram et al., 2010). The interrelation of social factors in the community and the structures of care provision has been the focus of this book.

The shocking fact of needless maternal death has become a strategic place from which to lobby for better care. But at the centre of my research was life, not death: the ordinary practices that made up the everyday lives of rural women seeking care. My research goal was to map the social organization of childbirth and maternity care in Amuru subcounty, northern Uganda. I listened to the narratives of mothers and health care workers, and paid attention to how health care provision and social conditions in the community informed maternity care and childbirth practices. IE works to capture how daily life is made up of activities, texts, and ideas that are observable within a local context but are also organized by ruling relations that are often extra-local in nature. This methodological approach helped me to see transnational influences within this remote rural setting. The landscape of care has also been shaped by the past LRA conflict, the current context of rebuilding in northern Uganda, and inadequate public resources. As the first study to focus on community-level childbirth and maternity care in this area since armed hostilities ended, a contribution of this research has been to offer empirical evidence that responds to a significant call for context-specific research on maternity care (Kyomuhendo, 2003; MacKian, 2008; Say & Raine, 2007; Spangler, 2011). This local context, it turned out, was enmeshed with global health discourses and practices that originated across the world and in the very different contexts of bureaucratic meetings and international cooperation.

Here, I provide an overview of the major findings and reflect on discursive practices that shape global health initiatives. This analysis of how global health approaches, including the MDGs, international NGOs, and shifting policy governing TBAs, shaped care in a remote community is a contribution that can be extended to develop our understanding of the dynamics within other health care settings struggling with maternal health.

## Global Goals, Local Lives

Throughout this book, I have focused on the interplay between material conditions, health care provision, and the operations of power. These central themes incorporate an emphasis on how the post-conflict context and lack of access to resources shaped how and where women accessed care. Macro-scale contexts such as global health policies, goals, and funding shaped care, as did micro-scale concerns such as household finances, relationships, and home location; this interplay informs my discussion of the continuing role of TBAs; the impact of the mama kits, a material resource distributed by NGOs; and the impact of compulsory, sometimes punitive, approaches to couples' HIV testing. To understand how practices are informed, I have examined the relevant policies and have paid special attention to tracking discourses – including those about people and place, and those about care and death. These discourses include representations that are problematic in terms of how they reference culture, difference, and choice. The movement between local and global and between material and discursive has been facilitated by institutional ethnographic methodologies, which help to tease apart the complex social organization of everyday activities. The approach that "data are everywhere" offers a freedom to pursue ideas and leads, adding new questions or new sites of inquiry as they become relevant.

The past LRA conflict and current post-conflict setting imposed individual and material hardships that have affected maternity care and childbirth. The conflict affected gender dynamics and work responsibilities and contributed to poverty and lack of access to resources. Armed conflict, abduction, and internment in IDP camps have caused individual and social traumas, which have in turn altered social relationships. Altered gender dynamics affect men's and women's activities in relation to pregnancy and birth, and some participants struggled with men's reluctance to attend ANC or assist with work. For participants who were raising the children of a deceased relative, or whose husbands had been disabled in the conflict and could not work, or in some cases both, these circumstances added to the workload of managing pregnancy and related health care. This was the case for Betty, who was raising 10 children, some born to a relative who had died during the conflict, with her husband, himself badly injured. Neither partner was able to adhere to medical advice to rest, and ensuring nutrition was difficult; such social realities affect the applicability of advice from health care workers on managing a healthy pregnancy.

Land disputes were a major concern, contributing to ongoing social and economic insecurity. For example, Anita's story about how her husband had been jailed for poaching on land that they saw as their community's demonstrates how land, livelihood, and political insecurity are linked. With her husband in jail, Anita struggled with providing for her two children and coping with the costs of another pregnancy. As the immediate aftermath of war settles, land disputes remain common, particularly those between individuals and larger organizations such as government and industry. Because of poverty and a lack of resources, childbearing women organized their approaches to care and birth around factors such as avoiding arduous work, ensuring adequate nutrition, and arranging transportation. These social factors, outside the health care system, were nevertheless influential on how women managed their pregnancy care.

In every conversation I had with women I learned about the arduous and complex work they undertook to care for their health and to access health care. This began with trying to eat well and rest, this simple advice becoming complicated for most participants for financial reasons. The work of pregnancy also included coordinating and saving for transportation to and from antenatal and delivery care, managing their husbands' participation in HIV testing during ANC, and coordinating supplies for a safe delivery and for newborn care. I came to understand the time, effort, and money pregnant women had to spend on coordinating access to the most basic resources primarily in terms of power. Lack of infrastructure and resources in the post-conflict setting, an authoritative and at times coercive approach to health care provision, and patriarchal power within marriages coalesced to diminish the ease with which women could care for their pregnancies and access maternity health care. Within IE, work is understood to be an intentional activity that "is done in some actual place under definite conditions and with definite resources, and it takes time" (Smith, 2005, p. 154). This study's investigation of the conditions under which, and resources with which, childbearing women undertook health work during pregnancy and birth demonstrates the impacts of power inequities in adding to this workload.

The transnational focus on promoting skilled attendance at birth was necessary, but various social factors coalesced to make it insufficient to the contexts of pregnancy in Amuru. Gender, poverty, and aspects of the social context shaped by the past conflict and the post-conflict setting are implicated in the organization of maternity care and birth, yet they frequently seem to be overlooked. People's experiences during the conflict affected how they approached care and their concerns about pregnancy and birth. Some women's experience of the war led them to worry about the visitation of bad spirits during pregnancy or labour, while women who had abdominal or genital injuries resulting from being shot or surviving a fire expressed their fears of miscarriage or other complications. Amid the overcrowding and under-protection, IDP camp residents did have access to formal health care. This access helped familiarize residents with such care, but access was removed for those who relocated to faraway homes once the camps were disbanded. On the other hand, lay care was the norm for those who had lived in the community during the conflict, because it was too dangerous to travel to health care facilities. Even for abductees, health care challenges existed alongside the many hardships of isolation, constant movement, and captivity. For pregnant women and for health care workers, these factors made accelerating skilled attendance at birth more difficult.

Transportation was one of the most complex logistical challenges pregnant women faced. Participants noted that access to the health centre for ANC or delivery was significantly impacted by the cost and availability of transportation, as well as by the time of day, the weather, the season, and cell phone reception. Transportation problems overlapped with another challenge, the fact that facilities within the sub-county that should have been able to support ANC and labour care were not actually equipped to do so. Had such facilities been operational at their designated levels, travel distances would have been shorter and more manageable, since women would not have had to make the longer trip to an operational health facility. The transportation challenge is then partially, perhaps primarily, a health services problem. Gaps in service provision and transportation challenges that were exacerbated by past conflict and the limited rebuilding of infrastructure disproportionately affected families living far from the operational health centre and trading (market) centre of Amuru. The disproportionate access challenges faced by women in remote communities that I observed in Amuru is a common pattern (Munjanja et al., 2012, p. 140).

The ability to access transportation to health centres impacted whether or not women gave birth at home with the assistance of a TBA. International, national, and local approaches to maternity care discourage the attendance of TBAs, although the practice has not been officially banned. At the international level, there has been a shift away from TBA training and towards the promotion of relying on SBAs (Say & Raine, 2007; Wirth et al., 2008). Nationally, there have been announcements of a ban against TBAs and other public announcements discouraging TBAs' practice (as discussed in chapter 3). In reifying SBAs and their precedence over TBAs, issues such as the quality and cultural appropriateness of care are often sidelined. Meanwhile, locally, TBAs have been encouraged to refer women to a health centre rather than attend births in their villages. (In my field notes, I observed, "If TBAs can't attend births, they need a new name!") Despite the policy preference for facility-based delivery, health care administrators in Amuru sub-county have recognized that some women will inevitably give birth at home because of limited health services, poor transportation, or other conditions. Administrators therefore made the case that it was preferable to have a TBA in attendance rather than somebody without any birthing skills or nobody at all. TBAs have requested that some supports be provided to allow them to offer services in ways that are safer for them and for birthing women. These modest supports were not, however, provided, as programming for TBAs was seen as antithetical to promoting skilled attendance at birth.

Instead of preference, the mothers who I interviewed associated their TBA-attended births with the inability to reach a health care facility. This is particularly significant given that several studies have associated reliance on TBAs with cultural preference (Ensor & Cooper, 2004; Izugbara et al., 2009; Montagu et al., 2011; Vallières et al., 2013). For example, a systematic review of qualitative studies on women's perceptions of obstetric services reported that "the mistrust of the modern healthcare system, coupled with a cultural preference for traditional medicine, leads to preferential use of TBAs" (Brighton et al., 2013, p. 225). Such findings often generate recommendations that are related to education and other "demand-side" interventions (Ensor & Cooper, 2004; Konde et al., 2011), including most recently a preponderance of funding and interest in apps for pregnant women in various settings. A focus on demand-side interventions suggests that the onus is on patients to do more to seek out quality care. Supporting women's knowledge of pregnancy-related health and health care will always be valuable; however, a demand-side focus can be problematic if it detracts from attention to the lack of quality care options available. Since, in Amuru, barriers to accessing formal care shaped both where and under whose care birth took place, there is a need for increased attention to accessible rural health care, using a nuanced understanding of access, rather than focusing on cultural preference. To the extent that high maternal mortality rates and other poor outcomes coincide with weak health care systems, it is worth keeping this dynamic front of mind in considerations of maternity health care in other similar settings.

The dynamics surrounding the mama kit NGO project were particularly illustrative of how local and translocal ideas and practices could clash and lead to dysfunction. When used to promote attendance at delivery, they became one site of the single-minded fixation on skilled attendance at birth. The relationship between mama kits and women's care-seeking practices was complex. While the kits were useful and valued, registration and distribution practices impacted maternity care in ways that had not been adequately considered. This was evident in the way that mama kit registration and distribution governed how care was sought, accessed, and delivered. The manner in which kits were distributed exemplified how strategies of scarcity led to competition for resources among childbearing women and inequitable access, both to these resources and to maternity care.

Women faced many hurdles on the way to a safe delivery. One aspect of ANC provision, couples' HIV testing, was a site of responsibilization for both women and men. In responsibilization, "the weight of responsibility for health is borne by the individual, rather than larger social structures and institutions" (Rossiter, 2012, p. 180). As such, it is a practice supported by neoliberal approaches to care and often associated with the discourse of consumer choice (Brown & Baker, 2012; Davies & Burns, 2013; LeBesco, 2011; Mykhalovskiy & McCoy, 2002). When we speak of health and health care as something within the purview of each individual, it becomes easier to overlook inadequacies of health care provision. In this case, responsibilization occurred in tandem with a paternalistic and directive approach to testing, which did not include a rhetoric of choice, though it did assume agency on the part of women. Instead, women were expected to comply with top-down directives. The top-down approach and compulsory approach to couples' HIV testing also promoted responsibilization. The requirement that women bring their male partners for testing led some to fear being denied care, while male reluctance to participate raised concern over potential violence targeted at women. Couples' testing represented a discursive site where global and national policies were (imperfectly) translated into local practices. Men's HIV testing was treated as ancillary to women's ANC, and men were targeted through their pregnant partners, rather than as individuals or as a group. Given that the approach was compulsory, recruiting men via their partners was problematic. Responsibilization strategies were used to coordinate the behaviour of individual women and, by proxy, their partners, but not to address problems within the health care system or structural factors that affect care.

## Discourses Governing Care: Choice, Tradition, and Culture

One place that standardizing and colonizing tendencies manifest is in a focus on barriers to access to care and on cultural preference, also labelled as *tradition*. As Kumar (2013) has argued, prioritizing technological solutions often means a turning away from structural causes, including structural violence (p. 25). The framing of the maternal health challenge as comprising access barriers plus cultural norms fails to adequately account for the institutional practices that produce the politics and practices of maternity care, practices that are simultaneously transnational and highly localized in scope. When maternity care studies rely on an analysis of choice and preference, the focus is on the individual or on what are held to be community norms. Concepts like choice and preference, however, are insufficient for theorizing why women rely on the people and places they do during maternity care and birth, or for mapping structural constraints. Instead of the objectifying approach of attributing poor outcomes to preferences shaped by "culture" and "tradition," it is necessary to look up and out from local contexts of care and investigate how they interact with broader contexts, including health systems, funding, and policies. In this way, the ruling relations that organize care can be understood. Highly specific and localized accounts of maternity care challenges, such as this research, have the potential to contribute to refining global health approaches to better meet the needs of parturient women in the global south.

The conversation on the maternal health crisis should not remain stalled at a focus on (technical) barriers to care and cultural preference surrounding care providers. Discussions of barriers and preferences often fail to adequately account for the social and institutional practices that produce the local politics of maternity care. Kumar (2013) identifies that "focusing on proximal determinants of health, such as access to healthcare, without giving due consideration to distal factors such as poverty and economic exploitation on a global and/or national scale" can be a form of colonial representation (p. 22). The impact of distal, or non-immediate, factors means that health care access should not be viewed primarily as a technical solution to maternal health problems in the global south; rather, it is important to also attend to structural factors, those that shape distal factors (Kumar, 2013, p. 25). The IE understanding of institutions as "a complex of ruling relations … that are organized around a particular function such as healthcare or education" (Smith, 1987) avoids a shift in analysis from social dimensions to technological dimensions of a problem, in this case the social organization of maternity care and birth. A focus on birth and maternity care as a social – rather than primarily technical and individual – process contributed to my understanding of how the organization of maternity care and birth is discursively produced through local networks and extra-local power relations.

The social dimension of maternity care and birth, however, should not be conflated with culture, despite the disproportionate reliance on culture as an explanatory concept in the literature on maternal health in global south settings. Instead, I see the social context of care as made up of the everyday work, activities, texts, and talk that pregnant women and health care workers enact in coordinating care. I am cautious of employing notions of "culture," or related concepts such as difference and tradition, as explanatory for how groups of women approach maternity care and birth. Approaches to care are dynamic rather than static and are coordinated by factors that cannot be reduced to culture. Therefore, while a thorough and nuanced understanding of local context, including cultural ideas or practices related to pregnancy and birth, is invaluable to understanding and improving maternity care, it is simultaneously necessary to be wary of deploying culture as a catch-all excuse for poor outcomes in particular settings. In "Writing Against Culture," anthropologist Lila Abu-Lughod (1991) argues that, in anthropology, the term *culture* operates "to enforce separations that inevitably carry a sense of hierarchy" (p. 466). In making the case against "culture," she identifies three problems: culture assumes "coherence, timelessness, and discreteness" (p. 472). She thus suggests a focus on discourse and ethnographies of the particular as strategies of "writing against culture." Like Abu-Lughod, Julie Taylor (2007) makes the case that reifying culture contributes to "power over" scenarios, as she traces a biomedical discourse that posits culture as a site of blame for HIV/AIDS. She writes that the concept of "culture" "may more often than not involve assertions of 'difference' and the subtle enforcement of inequality between 'self' and 'other' through that difference" (Taylor, 2007, p. 973).

Rather than emphasizing culture as a basis for activities related to maternity care, I employed IE sites of analysis, including of work and talk, in seeking to describe how approaches to care were shaped. These activities are not only powerful constituents of social practices but also viable places to introduce changes. A focus on how culture shapes preference is associated with recommendations to educate childbearing women. An example of this is provided by the literature recommending education or demand-side interventions as a means by which to reduce reliance on TBAs. In contrast, this research focused on everyday work, talk, texts, and practices, and led to findings that demonstrate where the need for social and institutional change lies. In making the case *for* attention to culture and tradition, Nabacwa and colleagues (2015) argue that Uganda's legal and policy context for maternity care is robust but that insufficient attention is paid to the harms of cultural beliefs and practices. Their discussion of potentially harmful cultural practices among the Acholi and other northern groups, including the Karamajong, introduces a wide range of examples from nutrition to wound care and concludes that "in some cases the women fail to access lifesaving services during pregnancy, delivery and postnatal care" (p. 175). What such studies cannot capture, however, is the role that cultural practices play when adequate health care services *are* available – care that is sufficiently close to home, culturally appropriate, and high quality.

In the absence of adequate care options, attention to how culture guides decisions is misplaced. Cultural practices are not fixed. For example, the practice of keeping babies indoors for three to four days has been cited as hindering women's decision to seek formal care (Nabacwa et al., 2015); however, I was told by women who used the health centre that this practice is persisting in a modified form, so that this period is counted as beginning after the return home from delivery. When culture is identified as a cause of certain approaches to health care, there is an implicit suggestion that any given approach is entrenched in the local people. Uganda's roadmap for reducing maternal mortality acknowledges that weak care provision plays an important role, in a phrasing that is otherwise emblematic of using culture as a tool of blame, claiming that "the poor health seeking behaviour of women due to negative cultures, reliance on traditional medicines and heavy workload at the ANC clinics remain a challenge" (UMOH, 2006, pp. 15, 16). To better understand the social constitution of maternity care and birth, it is necessary to reframe the interaction between culture and care.

*Choice* and *preference* are frequently the loci of analysis for research on maternity and childbirth care, as well as policies governing care provision. For example, it is common practice to describe where, and under whose care, women give birth primarily as a choice. The rhetoric of choice can obfuscate how state and NGO forces operate to determine and limit health care access for women (Rebick, 1993). Rurality and illiteracy or low educational attainment can compound these access problems: "Constraining choice may be especially likely when clients are women, rural and relatively uneducated compared to health personnel" (Angotti et al., 2011, p. 313). The women I spoke with recounted experiences regarding the location of birth that suggest that framings such as *choice, preference,* or *decision making* misrepresent critical contextual factors in coordinating approaches to care, such as transportation, cost, and proximity to health facility. For the foregoing reasons, while the principle of choice remains important in health care, knowledge of where and under whose care women give birth is not reducible to the analysis of women's choices. For choice to be a meaningful lens, access to viable options needs to be present.

Media and research studies have sometimes framed birth at home in Uganda as refusal or reluctance on the part of childbearing women to engage with formal care, identified in the media as "shunning," as discussed in chapter 1. In some instances, the continued reliance on TBAs for labour support is described as an entrenched preference, as is birth location (see for example Akpabio et al., 2012). This framing of birth location as preference is not supported by my research; I found little evidence that women are either refusing services or reluctant to participate in formal care. When women gave birth outside a health facility, it was often despite their best efforts to secure access to delivery care. In fact, participants identified the health centre as the norm for birthing location among their "fellow women." This finding is consistent with Koblinsky et al.'s (2006) conclusion that "for those who do not access care, the argument that services are available to meet their needs but are underused because of reluctance on the part of women is unlikely in countries where mortality rates are high" (p. 8).

These questions about choice, preference, and culture are theoretical as well as empirical in nature. A narrative about maternal health that centres preference or reluctance is harmful when it leads to blaming women, their beliefs, or their culture for poor outcomes, meanwhile avoiding an examination of structural problems. The fact that health centres were widely accepted as a desirable location to deliver does not diminish the importance of community-based TBAs who provide care to their neighbours. However, it does suggest that interventions should not be based on cultures of care or women's reluctance to give birth at health care facilities, but on improving access to care. My research indicated that, in contrast to cultural preference, a lack of operational care facilities and the cost, lack of availability, and general difficulty of transportation to health care facilities were the most prominent issues facing women who gave birth at home.

While I have argued against the discourse that women "shun" care for cultural reasons as a discourse of blame, responsibilization, and inattention to structure, I have also been moved by the strength of Acholi culture surrounding birth. The particularities of birth practices shift with shifting infrastructure for health care and other factors, but birth remains at the heart of stories about family and self. This is clearly evident in the language of naming, as I was struck by about two weeks into my time in Acholiland, thumbing through a dictionary to learn some vocabulary:

In my dictionary, the list of names has many that are associated with birth order or position. For example, "Acaa (f): From the noun 'kicaa.' It is given to a child born with the placenta membrane covering it. Acen (f): From the adverb 'cen' meaning behind. It is given to the second twin. Adoch (f): It is given to a child who comes out of the womb leg first. Akumu (f): It is given to a child conceived before the mother has resumed menstruation after the birth of the prior child. Alur (f): From the noun 'lur,' meaning barrenness. It is given to a child born to a woman/man who was thought to be barren/sterile." Lots about first/second twins, children born first or second after twins ... Also, "Atim, a child born in a foreign land or in the bush. Lamwaka: a child born at the end of the year/new year or after remaining in the womb for a full year. Lawino: From 'wino,' meaning placenta. It is given to a child when during its birth the placenta gets stuck in the mother's uterus. Acellum (m): The phrase means one child isn't enough. It is given to an only child." Lots around children born after other children's deaths. "Odoch (m): It is given to a child who comes out of the womb feet first instead of head first" (same as Adoch). Also to girls among boys, boys among girls. "Okot: From the noun 'kot,' which means rain. It is given to a child born with watery umbilical cords. Opiro: From the noun 'opiro,' which means sack or bag. It is given to children who are born inside the placenta and it is torn from outside the womb." Also for children born on the road.

It is a pleasure to meet Acholi people and to be able to guess a little of their birth story by their name. Together, the naming practices offer a sense of birth in Acholi as complex – those 12-month pregnancies and unexpected pregnancies – and with lifelong meaning to all family members. Babies are full members of the family: at school, where his classmates were being taught English, my son learned how to greet someone properly: "How are you? How is your father? How is your mother? How is the small baby, down in your home?" (Field note, May 9, 2012). Culture is not a problem to be overcome.

## Limitations

While the fieldwork of this study was still in progress, changes were being implemented that might ultimately impact maternity care and birth, but I did not have the opportunity to assess them. Of particular note was Lacor HCIII Amuru's plan to implement a one-time fee for pregnant women accessing ANC and delivery service. This fee was being levied in the final month of my fieldwork, and health care workers I spoke to suggested that the cost was too minimal to be a barrier or deterrent to women. The fee was low but might nevertheless present a barrier to those already struggling with the costs of preparation for birth and the new baby. By 2019, USAID was offering a voucher system, registered via the VHT, to assist vulnerable women with the fees. Assessing the introduction of fees and the subsequent introduction of a voucher system is beyond this study's scope, although it was notable that vulnerability was still a criterion and that the work for both patients and health workers was increased via the voucher system, as a maternity care staff person shared. It seems that some of the issues with the mama kits might arise within such a system. By 2019, roads had improved, shortening emergency transportation from the health centre to the hospital; while the blessings brought by roads are necessarily mixed, this was a positive change for access to emergency obstetrics, but one that I was unable to fully assess. The way care is provided is not static, and changes to staffing, facilities, and so on, impact the social organization of maternity care and birth.

Representation can be challenging. At times I have struggled to foreground the social organization of care without obscuring the hard work, commitment, and compassion of many of the health workers providing maternity care. Atul Gawande (2013), writing in *The New Yorker*, expresses a similar dilemma:

> Even the youngest nurses had done more than a thousand child deliveries. They've seen and learned to deal with countless problems – a torn placenta, an umbilical cord wrapped around a baby's neck, a stuck shoulder. Seeing the daily heroism required to keep such places going, you feel foolish and ill-mannered asking how they could do things better. (para. 22)

While I have been necessarily critical about the organization of care, I acknowledge the dedication and work of care providers. In my conversations with TBAs, their pride in and commitment to their work was evident. They shared the accomplishments of children at whose births they had assisted years before, telling me that one was attending university in the capital, or that another was now a mother herself. When I closed my interview with Amy by asking if there was anything that she needed to add, she told me about her journey to become first a nurse aide and then a nursing assistant. She said that as an orphan of the war, it had been a challenge to complete her education, and she finally had to stop on completing senior four (equivalent to junior high school or to an O-level). She had worked as a nursery teacher but felt called to serve as a nurse, and applied to the nurse aide position about 10 times. She told me: "And then at last I got that job. And I am so proud of it. And whenever a patient, a woman, wants help from me, I will give it so gladly. I give it gladly." While the commitment and working challenges of health care workers have not been my focus, I hope my respect for their work is evident.

## Conclusion

Extrapolating from the case of northern Uganda to the larger issue of how global health discourses and practices typically frame the crisis in maternal health and its solutions, the various failures and challenges identified throughout this book should not be seen as isolated or unusual; many are emblematic of global health dynamics. Adams (2010) argues that global health can act as "a new technology of governance in a post-colonial world" (p. 41), regulating recipients through health interventions. Kumar (2013) traces how qualitative research on birth in the global south has tended to reproduce objectifying colonial representations of childbearing women, while at the same time largely overlooking inequitable social relations resulting in "poverty and economic exploitation" (p. 22). These twin tendencies, to govern via large-scale standardized public health interventions shaped by global north technocracies while blaming local culture, tradition, and social relations for poor health outcomes, are pervasive within research and practice on the maternal health crisis in global south countries with high ratios of maternal mortality.

Social contexts, including poverty and post-conflict rebuilding, are not just a backdrop to but an essential part of what organizes maternity care and approaches to birth. Power relations and social justice issues are important considerations when planning care. Dying in childbirth is *not* part of any culture. Researchers and members of the health care sector need to accord respect to birthing women when thinking about where and under whose supervision they give birth. While health education efforts remain important, childbearing women also should be recognized as competent and knowledgeable when it comes to their own care needs.

# References


Abe, S. K., Murakami, Y., Morgan, D., & Shibuya, K. (2015). Rethinking the global tracking system on development assistance to reproductive, maternal, newborn, and child health. *The Lancet Global Health, 3*(7), E350–E351. https://doi.org/10.1016/S2214-109X(15)00043-1

Abu-Lughod, L. (2013). Writing against culture. In H. L. Moore & T. Sanders (Eds.), *Anthropology in theory: Issues in epistemology* (pp. 466–479). John Wiley & Sons. (Original work published 1991)

Achadi, E., Pitchforth, E., & Hussein, J. (2012). Quality of care. In J. Hussein, A. McCaw-Binns, & R. Webber (Eds.), *Maternal and perinatal health in developing countries* (pp. 181–192). CABI International.

Acholi MPs link nodding disease to weapons used during the war. (2012, May 21). *Acholi Times.* Retrieved January 15, 2014, from http://acholitimes.com/index.php/news/archives/8-acholi-news/366-acholi-mps-link-nodding-disease-to-weapons-used-during-the-warp

Ackers, L., Ioannou, E., & Ackers-Johnson, J. (2016). The impact of delays on maternal and neonatal outcomes in Ugandan public health facilities: the role of absenteeism. *Health Policy and Planning, 31*(9), 1152–1161. https://doi.org/10.1093/heapol/czw046

Adams, V. (2010). Against global health? Arbitrating science, non-science, and nonsense through health. In J. M. Metzl & A. Kirkland (Eds.), *Against health: How health became the new morality.* NYU Press.

Adyanga, A. F. (2012, March 8). A Ugandan (Acholi) perspective on Joseph Kony and Stop Kony 2012. *Eric's Wanderings.* http://ericswanderings.wordpress.com/2012/03/08/a-ugandan-acholi-perpective-on-joseph-kony-and-stop-kony-2012/

*Agreement on cessation of hostilities between the government of the Republic of Uganda and the Lord's Resistance Army/Movement, Juba, Sudan.* (2006, August 26). Peace Agreements. https://www.peaceagreements.org/viewmasterdocument/262

Ahimbisibwe, C. (2004, September 9). Pregnant women shun hospitals. *New Vision*. http://allafrica.com/stories/200409090135.html

Ahumuza, S. E., Rujumba, J., Nkoyooyo, A., Byaruhanga, R., & Wanyenze, R. K. (2016). Challenges encountered in providing integrated HIV, antenatal and postnatal care services: A case study of Katakwi and Mubende districts in Uganda. Reproductive Health, *13*, Article 41. https://doi.org /10.1186/s12978-016-0162-8

Akpabio, I. I., Edet, O. B., Etifit, R. E., & Robinson-Bassey, G. C. (2012). Preferences for traditional or modern practitioners: a comparative study. *African Journal of Midwifery and Women's Health, 6*(1), 13–20. https://doi .org/10.12968/ajmw.2012.6.1.13

Akumu, C. O., Amony, I., & Otim, G. (2005). *Suffering in silence: A study of sexual and gender based violence (SGBV) in Pabbo camp Gulu district northern Uganda*. Gulu District Sub Working Group on SGBV. https://reliefweb.int /sites/reliefweb.int/files/resources/BEFB77D29CC17FE74925702200095601 -unicef-uga-15jun.pdf

Allen, T. (2007). The International Criminal Court and the invention of traditional justice in Northern Uganda. *Politique Africaine, 107*(3), 147–166. https://doi.org/10.3917/polaf.107.0147

Amony, E. (2015). *I am Evelyn Amony: Reclaiming my life from the Lord's Resistance Army* (E. Baines, Ed.). University of Wisconsin Press.

Amony, E., & Shaya, T. (2012, November 27). *Agents of change: How war-affected women are advocating for change in Northern Uganda*. Open Canada. https:// opencanada.org/agents-of-change/

Amooti-Kaguna, B., & Nuwaha, F. (2000). Factors influencing choice of delivery sites in Rakai district of Uganda. *Social Science of Medicine, 50*(2), 203–213. https://doi.org/10.1016/S0277-9536(99)00275-0

Ana, J. (2011). Are traditional birth attendants good for improving maternal and perinatal health? Yes. *BMJ, 342*. https://doi.org/10.1136 /bmj.d3310

Anastasi, E., Borchert, M., Campbell, O. M. R., Sondorp, E., Kaducu, F., Hill, O., Okeng, D., Odong, V. N., & Lange, I. L. (2015). Losing women along the path to safe motherhood: why is there such a gap between women's use of antenatal care and skilled birth attendance? A mixed methods study in northern Uganda. *BMC Pregnancy and Childbirth, 15*(1), 287. https://doi.org /10.1186/s12884-015-0695-9

Angotti, N., Dionne, K. Y., & Gaydosh, L. (2011). An offer you can't refuse: Provider initiated HIV testing in Malawi. *Health Policy and Planning, 26*(4), 307–315. https://doi.org/10.1093/heapol/czq066

Annan, J., Blattman, C., Mazurana, D., & Carlson, K. (2011). Civil war, reintegration, and gender in Northern Uganda. *Journal of Conflict Resolution, 55*(6), 877–908. https://doi.org/10.1177/0022002711408013

Annan, J., & Brier, M. (2010). The risk of return: Intimate partner violence in Northern Uganda's armed conflict. *Social Science and Medicine, 70*(1), 152–159. https://doi.org/10.1016/j.socscimed.2009.09.027

Attaran, A. (2005). An immeasurable crisis? A criticism of the millennium development goals and why they cannot be measured. *PLoS Medicine, 2*(10), e318. https://doi.org/10.1371/journal.pmed.0020318

Austin, J., Guy, S., Lee-Jones, L., McGinn, T., & Schlecht, J. (2008). Reproductive health: A right for refugees and internally displaced persons. *Reproductive Health Matters, 16*(31), 10–21. https://doi.org/10.1016/S0968 -8080(08)31351-2

Baines, E. K. (2009). Complex political perpetrators: Reflections on Dominic Ongwen. *The Journal of Modern African Studies, 47*(2), 163–191.

Baines, E. K. (2012, March 12). *#Ugandans 2012.* Open Canada. https:// opencanada.org/ugandans2012/

Baines, E. K. (2014). Forced marriage as a political project: Sexual rules and relations in the Lord's Resistance Army. *Journal of Peace Research, 51*(3), 405–417. https://doi.org/10.1177/0022343313519666

Baines, E. K. (2017). *Buried in the heart: Women, complex victimhood and the war in northern Uganda.* Cambridge Univiersity Press.

Baines, E. K., & Rosenoff Gauvin, L. (2014). Motherhood and social repair after war and displacement in northern Uganda. *Journal of Refugee Studies, 27*(2), 282–300. https://doi.org/10.1093/jrs/feu001

Baines, E. K., & Stewart, B. (2011). "I cannot accept what I have not done": Storytelling, gender and transitional justice. *Journal of Human Rights Practice, 3*(3), 245–263. https://doi.org/10.1093/jhuman/hur015

Barnabas, O. D. (2013). Tragedy of the commons: From victims of Lord's Resistance Army conflict to victims of land conflicts. *Universal Journal of Education and General Studies, 2*(1), 15–20.

Barros, F. C., Matijasevich, A., Harris Requejo, J., Giugliani, E., Goretti Maranhão, A., Monteiro, C. A., Barros, A. J. D., Bustreo, F., Merialdi, M., & Victora, C. G. (2010). Recent trends in maternal, newborn, and child health in brazil: Progress toward millennium development goals 4 and 5. *American Journal of Public Health, 100*(10), 1877–1889. https://doi.org/10.2105/AJPH .2010.196816

Benton, A. (2015). *HIV exceptionalism: Development through disease in Sierra Leone.* University of Minnesota Press.

Biehl, J., & Petryna, A. (2013). Critical global health. In J. Biehl & A. Petryna (Eds.), *When people come first: Critical studies in global health* (pp. 1–20). Princeton University Press.

Bisaillon, L. (2012). An analytic glossary to social inquiry using institutional and political activist ethnography. *International Journal of Qualitative Methods, 11*(5), 607–627. https://doi.org/10.1177/160940691201100506

Bitek, J. O. (2012). A chronology of compassion, or towards an imperfect future. *International Journal of Transitional Justice, 6*(3), 394–403. https://doi.org/10.1093/ijtj/ijs021

Branch, A. (2011). *Displacing human rights: War and intervention in northern Uganda.* Oxford University Press.

Branch, A. (2012). *Challenges for human rights defenders in northern Uganda* [Speech. transcript]. Human Rights Focus. https://hurifo.ug/wp-content/uploads/Examiner//examiner1_2012.pdf

Branch, A. (2013). Gulu in war … and peace? The town as camp in Northern Uganda. *Urban Studies, 50*(15), 3152–3167. https://doi.org/10.1177/0042098013487777

Brighton, A., D'Arcy, R., Kirtley, S., & Kennedy, S. (2013). Perceptions of prenatal and obstetric care in Sub-Saharan Africa. *International Journal of Gynecology & Obstetrics,* 120(3), 224–227. https://doi.org/10.1016/j.ijgo.2012.09.017

Brown, B. J., & Baker, S. (2012). *Responsible citizens: Individuals, health, and policy under neoliberalism.* Anthem Press.

Browne, A. J., Smye, V. L., & Varcoe, C. (2005). The relevance of postcolonial theoretical perspectives to research in Aboriginal health. *Canadian Journal of Nursing Research,* 37(4), 16–37. PMID: 16541817

Butler, J. (2015). *Notes toward a performative theory of assembly.* Harvard University Press.

Campbell, M. L., & Gregor, F. M. (2002). *Mapping social relations: A primer in doing institutional ethnography.* Rowman Altamira.

Campbell, M. L., & Teghtsoonian, K. (2010). Aid effectiveness and women's empowerment: Practices of governance in the funding of international development. *Signs: Journal of Women in Culture and Society, 36*(1), 177–202. https://doi.org/10.1086/652914

Campbell, O., & Graham, W. (2006). Strategies for reducing maternal mortality: Getting on with what works. *Lancet,* 368(9543), 1284–1299. https://doi.org/10.1016/S0140-6736(06)69381

Center for Health, Human Rights and Development. (2012). *Strategic litigation programme.* https://www.cehurd.org/programmes/strategic-litigation/

Chan, J. (2015). *Politics in the corridor of dying: AIDS activism and global health governance.* John Hopkins University Press.

Chi, P. C., Bulage, P., Urdal, H., & Sundby, J. (2015a). Perceptions of the effects of armed conflict on maternal and reproductive health services and outcomes in Burundi and Northern Uganda: A qualitative study. *BMC International Health and Human Rights, 15*(1), 7. https://doi.org/10.1186/s12914-015-0045-z

Chi, P. C., Bulage, P., Urdal, H., & Sundby, J. (2015b). Barriers in the delivery of emergency obstetric and neonatal care in post-conflict Africa:

Qualitative case studies of Burundi and Northern Uganda. *PLoS One, 10*(9). https://doi.org/10.1371/journal.pone.0139120

Conrad, P., De Allegri, M., Moses, A., Larsson, E. C., Neuhann, F., Müller, O., & Sarker, M. (2012). Antenatal care services in rural Uganda: Missed opportunities for good-quality care. *Qualitative Health Research, 22*(5), 619–629. https://doi.org/10.1177/1049732311431897

Corbin, J. N. (2008). Returning home: Resettlement of formerly abducted children in Northern Uganda. *Disasters, 32*(2), 316–335. https://doi.org/10.1111/j.0361-3666.2008.01042.x

Coulter, J. B. S. (2001). Dr Matthew Lukwiya, medical superintendent, St Mary's Hospital, Lacor, Uganda, died of Ebola virus, December 2000. *Annals of Tropical Paediatrics, 21*(2), 101–103. https://doi.org/10.1080/02724930120058142

Cowley, D. (2013). Lucille Teasdale. In *The Canadian Encyclopedia*. Retrieved January 15, 2020, from https://www.thecanadianencyclopedia.ca/en/article/lucille-teasdale

Crane, J. T. (2013). *Scrambling for Africa: AIDS, expertise, and the rise of American global health science.* Cornell University Press.

Crenshaw, K. (1991). Mapping the margins: Intersectionality, identity politics, and violence against women of color. *Stanford Law Review, 43*(6), 1241–1299. https://doi.org/10.2307/1229039

Das, P., & Horton, R. (2018). Beyond the silos: Integrating HIV and global health. *The Lancet, 392*(10144), 260–261. https://doi.org/10.1016/S0140-6736(18)31466-1

Davies, C., & Burns, K. (2013). Mediating healthy female citizenship in the HPV vaccination campaigns. *Feminist Media Studies, 14*(5), 711–726. https://doi.org/10.1080/14680777.2013.830632

*Declaration of Alma-Ata.* (1978). International Conference on Primary Health Care, Alma-Ata, USSR, 6–12 September 1978. https://www.who.int/publications/almaata_declaration_en.pdf

DeVault, M. L., & McCoy, L. (2006). Institutional ethnography: Using interviews to investigate ruling relations. In D. Smith (Ed.), *Institutional ethnography as practice* (pp. 15–44). Rowman & Littlefield.

Devi, S. (2014). Uganda takes "another step backward" with HIV bill. *The Lancet, 383*(9933), 1960. https://doi.org/10.1016/s0140-6736(14)60941-7

Dickinson, C., Attawell, K., & Druce, N. (2009). Progress on scaling up integrated services for sexual and reproductive health and HIV. *Bulletin of the World Health Organization, 87*, 846–851. https://doi.org/10.2471/BLT.08.059279

Dilger, H., & Mattes, D. (2018). Im/mobilities and dis/connectivities in medical globalisation: How global is global health? *Global Public Health, 13*(3), 265–275. https://doi.org/10.1080/17441692.2017.1414285

Dolan, C. (2009). *Social torture: The case of northern Uganda, 1986–2006* (Vol. 4). Berghahn Books.

Eaton, J. W., Rehle, T. M., Jooste, S., Nkambule, R., Kim, A. A., Mahy, M., & Hallett, T. B. (2014). Recent HIV prevalence trends among pregnant women and all women in sub-Saharan Africa: Implications for HIV estimates. *AIDS (London, England), 28*(4), S507–S514. https://doi.org /10.1097/QAD.0000000000000412

Ediau, M., Wanyenze, R. K., Machingaidze, S., Otim, G., Olwedo, A., Iriso, R., & Tumwesigye, N. M. (2013). Trends in antenatal care attendance and health facility delivery following community and health facility systems strengthening interventions in Northern Uganda. *BMC Pregnancy and Childbirth, 13*(189), 1–11. https://doi.org/10.1186/1471-2393-13-189

Emasu, A. (2006, October 30). Why K'jong women still shun the labour ward. *New Vision*. http://allafrica.com/stories/200610310156.html

Englert, E. G., Kiwanuka, R., & Neubauer, L. C. (2018). "When I die, let me be the last": Community health worker perspectives on past Ebola and Marburg outbreaks in Uganda. *Global Public Health, 14*(8), 1182–1192. https://doi.org/10.1080/17441692.2018.1552306

Ensor, T., & Cooper, S. (2004). Overcoming barriers to health service access: Influencing the demand side. *Health Policy and Planning, 19*(2), 69–79. https://doi.org/10.1093/heapol/czh009

Fabiani, M., Nattabi, B., Opio, A. A., Musinguzi, J., Biryahwaho, B., Ayella, E. O., Ogwang, M., & Declich, S. (2006). A high prevalence of HIV-1 infection among pregnant women living in a rural district of north Uganda severely affected by civil strife. *Transactions of The Royal Society of Tropical Medicine and Hygiene, 100*(6), 586–593. https://doi.org/10.1016/j.trstmh .2005.09.002

Falk, L., Lenz, J. A., & Okuma, P. (2004). *Sleepless in Gulu: A study of the dynamics behind the child night commuting phenomena in Gulu, Uganda*. Save the Children. https://resourcecentre.savethechildren.net/sites/default/files /documents/2373.pdf

Farmer, P. (2008). Challenging orthodoxies: The road ahead for health and human rights. *Health and Human Rights, 10*(1), 5–19. https://doi.org /10.2307/20460084

Farmer, P. (2010). *Partner to the poor: A Paul Farmer reader* (Vol. 23). University of California Press.

Filippi, V., Ronsmans, C., Campbell, O. M. R., Graham, W. J., Mills, A., Borghi, J., Koblinsky, M., & Osrin, D. (2006). Maternal health in poor countries: the broader context and a call for action. *The Lancet, 368*(9546), 1535–1541. https://doi.org/10.1016/S0140-6736(06)69384-7

Finnegan, A. C. (2013). The white girl's burden. *Contexts, 12*(1), 30–35. https://doi.org/10.1177/1536504213476243

Finnström, S. (2008). *Living with bad surroundings: War, history, and everyday moments in northern Uganda.* Duke University Press.

Fleming, P. J., Colvin, C., Peacock, D., & Dworkin, S. L. (2016). What role can gender-transformative programming for men play in increasing men's HIV testing and engagement in HIV care and treatment in South Africa? *Culture, Health & Sexuality, 18*(11), 1251–1264. https://doi.org/10.1080/13691058.2016.1183045

Foley, E. E. (2008). The anti-politics of health reform: Household power relations and child health in rural Senegal. *Anthropology & Medicine, 16*(1), 61–71. https://doi.org/10.1080/13648470802426243

Galtung, J. (1969). Violence, peace and peace research. *Journal of Peace Research, 6*(3), 167–191. https://doi.org/10.1177/002234336900600301

Gauvin, L. R. (2013). In and out of culture: Okot p'Bitek's work and social repair in post-conflict Acoliland. *Oral Tradition, 28*(1). https://doi.org/10.1353/ort.2013.0008

Gawande, A. (2013, July 29). Slow ideas. *New Yorker.* https://www.mainequalitycounts.org/image_upload/Slow%20Ideas%20-%20The%20New%20Yorker.pdf

Gilbert, E., & Otika, B. (2013). *Five health workers of Otwee Health Centre III in Amuru Town Council arrested over negligence of duty.* Retrieved January 15, 2014, from http://kic.wougnet.org

Gilson, E. C. (2018). Beyond bounded selves and places: The relational making of vulnerability and security. *Journal of the British Society for Phenomenology, 49*(3), 229–242. https://doi.org/10.1080/00071773.2018.1434972

Grace, D. (2013). Transnational institutional ethnography: Tracing text and talk beyond state boundaries. *International Journal of Qualitative Methods, 12*(1), 587–605. https://doi.org/10.1177/160940691301200131

Grace, D. (2015). Criminalizing HIV transmission using model law: Troubling best practice standardizations in the global HIV/AIDS response. *Critical Public Health, 25*(4), 441–454. https://doi.org/10.1080/09581596.2015.1049121

Grahame, P. R. (1998). Ethnography, institutions, and the problematic of the everyday world. *Human Studies, 21*(4), 347–360. https://doi.org/10.1023/A:1005469127008

Griffith, A. I., & Smith, D. E. (1987). Constructing cultural knowledge: Mothering as discourse. In J. S. Gaskell & A. Tiger McLaren (Eds.), *Women and education: A Canadian perspective* (pp. 87–104). Detselig Enterprises.

Hankivsky, O., Grace, D., Hunting, G., Ferlatte, O., Clark, N., Fridkin, A., Giesbrecht, M., Rudrum, S., & Laviolette, T. (2012). Intersectionality-based policy analysis. In O. Hankivsky (Ed.), *An intersectionality-based policy analysis framework* (pp. 33–45). Institute for Intersectionality Research and Policy; Simon Fraser University.

Hardon, A., Vernooij, E., Bongololo-Mbera, G., Cherutich, P., Desclaux, A., Kyaddondo, D., Ky-Zerbo, O., Neuman, M., Wanyenze, R., & Obermeyer, C. (2012). Women's views on consent, counseling and confidentiality in PMTCT: A mixed-methods study in four African countries. *BMC Public Health, 12*(26), 1–15. https://doi.org/10.1186/1471-2458-12-26

Harrison, K. A. (2011). Are traditional birth attendants good for improving maternal and perinatal health? *BMJ, 342*, d3308. https://doi.org/10.1136/bmj.d3308

Harvey, S. A., Ayabaca, P., Bucagu, M., Djibrina, S., Edson, W. N., Gbangbade, S., McCaw-Binns, A., & Burkhalter, B. R. (2004). Skilled birth attendant competence: an initial assessment in four countries, and implications for the Safe Motherhood movement. *International Journal of Gynecology & Obstetrics, 87*(2), 203–210. https://doi.org/10.1016/j.ijgo.2004.06.017

Hladik, W., Musinguzi, J., Kirungi, W., Opio, A., Stover, J., Kaharuza, F., Bunnell, R., Kafuko, J., & Mermin, J. (2008). The estimated burden of HIV/AIDS in Uganda, 2005–2010. *AIDS, 22*(4), 503–510. https://doi.org/10.1097/QAD.0b013e3282f470be

Horton, R. (2014). Offline: Why the Sustainable Development Goals will fail. *The Lancet, 383*(9936), 2196. https://doi.org/10.1016/S0140-6736(14)61046-1

Huby, G., Hart, E., McKevitt, C., & Sobo, E. (2007). Addressing the complexity of health care: The practical potential of ethnography. *Journal of Health Services Research & Policy, 12*(4), 193–194. https://doi.org/10.1258/135581907782101516

Hussey, I. (2012). "Political activist as ethnographer" revisited. *Canadian Journal of Sociology, 37*(1), 1–24. https://doi.org/10.29173/cjs10214

Ingram, A. (2013). After the exception: HIV/AIDS beyond salvation and scarcity. *Antipode, 45*(2), 436–454. https://doi.org/10.1111/j.1467-8330.2012.01008.x

Institute for Health Metrics and Evaluation. (2014). *Health service provision in Uganda: Assessing facility capacity, costs of care, and patient perspectives.*

Invisible Children. (2012). *Kony 2012.* http://invisiblechildren.com/kony/

Izugbara, C., Ezeh, A., & Fotso, J.-C. (2009). The persistence and challenges of homebirths: Perspectives of traditional birth attendants in urban Kenya. *Health Policy and Planning, 24*(1), 36–45. https://doi.org/10.1093/heapol/czn042

Jakubec, S. L., & Campbell, M. (2003). Mental health research and cultural dominance: The social construction of knowledge for international development. *Canadian Journal of Nursing Research Archive, 35*(2). PMID: 12908198

Janes, C. R., & Corbett, K. K. (2009). Anthropology and global health. *Annual Review of Anthropology, 38*, 167–183. https://doi.org/10.1146/annurev-anthro-091908-164314

Jokhio, A. H., Winter, H. R., & Cheng, K. K. (2005). An intervention involving traditional birth attendants and perinatal and maternal mortality in Pakistan. *New England Journal of Medicine, 352*(20), 2091–2099. https://doi.org/10.1056/NEJMsa042830

Kinsman, J. (2012). "A time of fear": Local, national, and international responses to a large Ebola outbreak in Uganda. *Globalization and Health, 8*(15), 1–12. https://doi.org/10.1186/1744-8603-8-15

Knudsen, L. (2003). Limited choices: A look at women's access to health care in Kiboga, Uganda. *Women's* Studies Quarterly, *31*(3/4), 253–260. https://doi.org/131.162.213.108

Koblinsky, M., Matthews, Z., Hussein, J., Mavalankar, D., Mridha, M. K., Anwar, I., Achadi, E., Adjei, S., Padmanabhan, P., Marchal, B., De Brouwere, V., van Lerberghe, W., & Lancet Maternal Survival Series Steering Group. (2006). Going to scale with professional skilled care. *The Lancet, 368*(9544), 1377–1386. https://doi.org/10.1016/S0140- 6736(06)69382–3

Kolyangha, M. (2011, September 16). Pallisa mothers shun antenatal care. *The Monitor.* http://allafrica.com/stories/201109160183.html

Konde, A., Dolamo, B. L., & Monareng, L. V. (2011). Ugandan women's childbirth preferences. *Africa Journal of Nursing and Midwifery, 13*(2), 3–13. https://doi.org/10.10520/EJC19381

Krause, M. (2014). *The good project: Humanitarian relief NGOs and the fragmentation of reason.* University of Chicago Press.

Kumar, R. (2013). How are women's experiences of childbirth represented in the literature? A critical review of qualitative health research set in the global south. *Women's* Health and Urban Life, *12*(1), 19–38. http://hdl.handle.net/1807/35220

Kyomugisha, H. (2008). Traditional medicine: Oversight of practitioners and practices in Uganda. *Telecommunications & Regulated Industries.* https://doi.org/10.2139/ssrn.1322093

Kyomuhendo, G. B. (2003). Low use of rural maternity services in Uganda: Impact of women's status, traditional beliefs and limited resources. *Reproductive Health Matters, 11*(21), 16–26. https://doi.org/10.1016/S0968-8080(03)02176-1

Kyomuhendo, G. B. (2004). Cultural and resource determinants of severe maternal morbidity: Lessons from some "near miss" experiences. *African Sociological Review, 8*(1), 67–82. https://www.ajol.info/index.php/asr/article/viewFile/23237/19923

Kyomuhendo, G. B. (2009). Culture, pregnancy and childbirth in Uganda: Surviving the women's battle. In H. Selin (Ed.), *Childbirth across cultures: Ideas and practices of pregnancy, childbirth and the postpartum* (pp. 229–234). Springer.

Lacey, M. (2003). Nodding disease: Mystery of southern Sudan. *The Lancet Neurology, 2*(12), 714. https://doi.org/10.1016/S1474-4422(03)00599-4

Lacor Hospital. (n.d.-a). *Humanitarian activities.* Retrieved January 17, 2018, from: http://www.lacorhospital.org/the-hospital/humanitarian-activities

Lacor Hospital. (n.d.-b). *Matthew Lukwiya.* Retrieved January 17, 2018 from: http://www.lacorhospital.org/the-hospital/dr-matthew-lukwiya/

Laing, T., & Weschler, S. (2018). *Displacement as resistance in Northern Uganda: government abuse, popular protest, and the limits of international governance.* London School of Economics and Political Science. http://eprints.lse .ac.uk/id/eprint/91892

Larsson, E. C., Thorson, A., Pariyo, G., Conrad, P., Arinaitwe, M., Kemigisa, M., Erikson, J., Tomson, G., & Ekström, A. M. (2012). Opt-out HIV testing during antenatal care: Experiences of pregnant women in rural Uganda. *Health Policy and Planning, 27*(1), 69–75. https://doi.org/10.1093/heapol /czr009

Lawino, S. (2012, April 21). Amuru women undress before Madhvani boss. *The Monitor.* Retrieved October 15, 2013, from http://www.monitor.co.ug /News/National/-/688334/1390386/-/avks9ez/-/index.html

LeBesco, K. (2011). Neoliberalism, public health, and the moral perils of fatness. *Critical Public Health, 21*(2), 153–164. https://doi.org/10.1080 /09581596.2010.529422

Levi-Strauss, C. (1965). The principle of reciprocity. In L. A. Coser & B. Rosenberg (Eds.), *Sociological theory* (pp. 74–84). McMillan.

Lincetto, O., Mothebesoane-Anoh, S., Gomez, P., & Munjanja, S. (2006). Opportunities to deliver newborn care in existing programmes. In J. Lawn & K. Kerber (Eds.), *Opportunities for Africa's newborns: Practical data, policy and programmatic support for newborn care in Africa* (pp. 35–151). Partnership for Maternal, Newborn & Child Health. https://www.who.int /pmnch/media/publications/oanfullreport.pdf

Livingston, J. (2012). *Improvising medicine: An African oncology ward in an emerging cancer epidemic.* Duke University Press.

Lowndes, R. (2012). *Diabetes care and serious mental illness: An institutional ethnography* [Doctoral dissertation]. University of Toronto, TSpace Repository. https://tspace.library.utoronto.ca/bitstream/1807/34789/1 /Lowndes_Ruth_H_201211_PhD_thesis.pdf

MacKian, S. C. (2008). What the papers say: Reading therapeutic landscapes of women's health and empowerment in Uganda. *Health & Place, 14*(1), 106–115. https://doi.org/10.1016/j.healthplace.2007.05.005

MacVicar, S., Berrang-Ford, L., Harper, S., Steele, V., Lwasa, S., Bambaiha, D. N., Twesigomwe, S., Asaasira, G., IHACC Research Team, & Ross, N. (2017). How seasonality and weather affect perinatal health: Comparing the experiences of Indigenous and non-Indigenous mothers in Kanungu District, Uganda. *Social Science & Medicine, 187,* 39–48. https://doi.org /10.1016/j.socscimed.2017.06.021

Mafaranga. (2013). *Uganda: Traditional birth attendants blamed for HIV among newborn babies.* All Africa. Retrieved January 15, 2014, from http://allafrica .com/stories/201312191063.html

Magnussen, L., Ehiri, J., & Jolly, P. (2004). Comprehensive versus selective primary health care: lessons for global health policy. *Health Affairs, 23*(3), 167–176. https://doi.org/10.1377/hlthaff.23.3.167

Malinga, J. (2010, June 30). Traditional birth attendants show no sign of abandoning their work in Katine. *The Guardian.* https://www.theguardian .com/katine/2010/jun/30/traditional-birth-attendants-work

Mannay, D., & Morgan, M. (2014). Doing ethnography or applying a qualitative technique? Reflections from the "waiting field." *Qualitative Research, 15*(2), 166–182. https://doi.org/10.1177/1468794113517391

Matsiko, C. W., & Kiwanuka, J. (2003). A review of human resource for health in Uganda. *Health Policy and Development, 1*(1), 15–20. http://hdl.handle .net/20.500.12280/1359

Mauss, M. (1990). *The gift* (W. D. Halls, Trans.). Routledge. (Original work published 1925)

Mawdsley, E. (2012). The changing geographies of foreign aid and development cooperation: contributions from gift theory. *Transactions of the Institute of British Geographers, 37*(2), 256–272. https://doi.org/10.1111 /j.1475-5661.2011.00467.x

Mazurana, D. E., McKay, S. A., Carlson, K. C., & Kasper, J. C. (2002). Girls in fighting forces and groups: Their recruitment, participation, demobilization, and reintegration. *Peace and Conflict: Journal of Peace Psychology, 8*(2), 97–123. https://doi.org/10.1207/S15327949PAC0802_01

Mbonye, A. K., Yanow, S., Birungi, J., & Magnussen, P. (2013). A new strategy and its effect on adherence to intermittent preventive treatment of malaria in pregnancy in Uganda. *BMC Pregnancy and Childbirth, 13*(178), 1–7. https://doi.org/10.1186/1471-2393-13-178

McCoy, L. (2006). Keeping the institution in view: Working with interview accounts of everyday experience. In D. E. Smith (Ed.), *Institutional ethnography as practice* (pp. 109–125). Rowman & Littlefield Publishers.

McElroy, T. (2012). *Early childhood before, during and after war and displacement in northern Uganda* [Doctoral dissertation]. University of British Columbia, Open Collections, UBC Theses and Dissertations. https://doi.org/10.14288 /1.0076895

McElroy, T., Muyinda, H., Atim, S., Spittal, P., & Backman, C. (2012). War, displacement and productive occupations in Northern Uganda. *Journal of Occupational Science, 19*(3), 198–212. https://doi.org/10.1080/14427591.2011.614681

Medley, A. M., Mugerwa, G. W., Kennedy, C., & Sweat, M. (2012). Ugandan men's attitudes toward their partner's participation in antenatal HIV testing. *Health Care for Women International, 33*(4), 359–374. https://doi.org/10.1080/07399332.2012.655392

Miller, S., Abalos, E., Chamillard, M., Ciapponi, A., Colaci, D., Comandé, D., Diaz, V., Geller, S., Hanson, C., Langer, A., Manuelli, V., Millar, K., Morhason-Bello, I., Pileggi Castro, C., Nogueira Pileggi, V., Robinson, N., Skaer, M., Paulo Souza, J., Vogel, J. P., & Althabe, F. (2016). Beyond too little, too late and too much, too soon: a pathway towards evidence-based, respectful maternity care worldwide. *The Lancet, 388*(10056), 2176–2192. https://doi.org/10.1016/S0140-6736(16)31472-6

Mitchell, K. B., Kornfeld, J., Adiama, J., Mugenyi, A., Schmutzhard, E., Ovuga, E., Kamstra, J., & Winkler, A. S. (2013). Nodding syndrome in northern Uganda: Overview and community perspectives. *Epilepsy & Behavior, 26*(1), 22–24. https://doi.org/10.1016/j.yebeh.2012.10.030

Mohanty, C. T. (1988). Under Western eyes: Feminist scholarship and colonial discourses. *Feminist Review, 30*, 61–88. https://doi.org/10.2307/1395054

Mohanty, C. T. (2013). Transnational feminist crossings: On neoliberalism and radical critique. *Signs, 38*(4), 967–991. https://doi.org/10.1086/669576

Montagu, D., Yamey, G., Visconti, A., Harding, A., & Yoong, J. (2011). Where do poor women in developing countries give birth? A multi-country analysis of demographic and health survey data. *PLoS ONE, 6*(2), e17155. https://doi.org/10.1371/journal.pone.0017155

Munabi-Babigumira, S., Glenton, C., Willcox, M., & Nabudere, H. (2019). Ugandan health workers' and mothers' views and experiences of the quality of maternity care and the use of informal solutions: A qualitative study. *PLoS ONE, 14*(3), e0213511. https://doi.org/10.1371/journal.pone.0213511

Munjanja, S. P., Magure, T., & Kandawasvika, G. (2012). Geographical access, transport and referral systems. In J. Hussein, A. McCaw-Binns, & R. Webber (Eds.), *Maternal and perinatal health in developing countries* (pp. 139–154). CABI

Murigi, S., & Ford, L. (2010, March 10). Should Uganda ban traditional birth attendants? *The Guardian.* https://www.theguardian.com/katine/katine-chronicles-blog/2010/mar/30/traditional-birth-attendants-ban

Muyinda, H., & Mugisha, J. (2015). Stock-outs, uncertainty and improvisation in access to healthcare in war-torn Northern Uganda. *Social Science & Medicine, 146*, 316–323. https://doi.org/10.1016/j.socscimed.2015.10.022

Mykhalovskiy, E., & McCoy, L. (2002). Troubling ruling discourses of health: Using institutional ethnography in community-based research. *Critical Public Health, 12*(1), 17–37. https://doi.org/10.1080/09581590110113286

Mykhalovskiy, E., McCoy, L., & Bresalier, M. (2004). Compliance/adherence, HIV, and the critique of medical power. *Social Theory & Health, 2*(4), 315–340. https://doi.org/10.1057/palgrave.sth.8700037

Nabacwa, M. S., Waiswa, J., Kabanda, M., Sentumbwe, O., & Anibaya, S. (2015). Culture, traditions and maternal health: A Community approach towards improved maternal health in the northern Uganda districts of Gulu, Moroto and Kotido. In *Millennium Development Goals (MDGs) in retrospect* (pp. 159–178). Springer, Cham.

Namasivayam, A., González, P. A., Delgado, R. C., & Chi, P. C. (2017). The effect of armed conflict on the utilization of maternal health services in Uganda: A population-based study. *PLoS Currents, 9.* https://doi.org/10.1371/currents.dis.557b987d6519d8c7c96f2006ed3c271a

Naulele, S. (2010). Kaberamaido mothers shun hospitals, *New Vision.* Retrieved January 15, 2014, from http://www.newvision.co.ug/PA/8/17/717596

Nussbaum, M. (2000). Women's capabilities and social justice. *Journal of Human Development, 1*(2), 219–247. https://doi.org/10.1080/713678045

Nussbaum, M. (2003). Capabilities as fundamental entitlements: Sen and social justice. *Feminist Economics, 9*(2–3), 33–59. https://doi.org/10.1080/1354570022000077926

O'Hare, B., & Southall, D. P. (2007). First do no harm: The impact of recent armed conflict on maternal and child health in Sub-Saharan Africa. *Journal of the Royal Society of Medicine, 100*(12), 564–570. https://doi.org/10.1177/0141076807100012015

Okello, M. C., & Hovil, L. (2007). Confronting the reality of gender-based violence in northern Uganda. *International Journal of Transitional Justice, 1*(3), 433–443. https://doi.org/10.1093/ijtj/ijm036

Omona, J., & Aduo, J. R. (2013). Gender issues during post-conflict recovery: The case of Nwoya district, northern Uganda. *Journal of Gender Studies, 22*(2), 119–136. https://doi.org/10.1080/09589236.2012.723359

Oosterom, M. (2011). Gender and fragile citizenship in Uganda: The case of Acholi women. *Gender & Development, 19*(3), 395–408. https://doi.org/10.1080/13552074.2011.625650

Owich, J. (2019). Uganda: Only 5 ambulances serve over 1M in Acholi. *The Monitor.* https://allafrica.com/stories/201905020635.html

Owor, A., & Dieterle, C. (2020, April 7). Customary land claims are at stake in northern Uganda. *Africa at LSE.* https://blogs.lse.ac.uk/africaatlse/2020/04/07/customary-land-claims-reform-unrecognised-in-northern-uganda/

Padian, N. S., McCoy, S. I., Karim, S. S., Hasen, N., Kim, J., Bartos, M., Katabira, E., Bertozzi, S. M., Schwartländer, B., & Cohen, M. S. (2011). HIV prevention transformed: The new prevention research agenda. *The Lancet, 378*(9787), 269–278. https://doi.org/10.1016/S0140-6736(11)60877-5

Pariyo, G. W., Mayora, C., Okui, O., Ssengooba, F., Peters, D. H., Serwadda, D., Lucas, H., Bloom, G., Rahman, M. H., & Ekirapa-Kiracho, E. (2011). Exploring new health markets: Experiences from informal providers of transport for maternal health services in Eastern Uganda. *BMC International Health and Human Rights, 11*(Suppl 1), S10. https://doi.org/10.1186/1472-698X-11-S1-S10

Parkhurst, J. O. (2011). Evidence, politics and Uganda's HIV success: Moving forward with ABC and HIV prevention. *Journal of International Development, 23*(2), 240–252. https://doi.org/10.1002/jid.1667

Parkhurst, J. O., Rahman, S. A., & Ssengooba, F. (2006). Overcoming access barriers for facility-based delivery in low-income settings: Insights from Bangladesh and Uganda. *Journal of Health, Population, and Nutrition, 24*(4), 438–445. https://www.ncbi.nlm.nih.gov/pmc/articles/PMC3001147/pdf/jhpn0024-0438.pdf

Patel, S., Schechter, M. T., Sewankambo, N. K., Atim, S., Lakor, S., Kiwanuka, N., & Spittal, P. M. (2014a). War and HIV: Sex and gender differences in risk behaviour among young men and women in post-conflict Gulu District, Northern Uganda. *Global Public Health, 9*(3), 325–341. https://doi.org/10.1080/17441692.2014.887136

Patel, S., Schechter, M. T., Sewankambo, N. K., Atim, S., Lakor, S., Kiwanuka, N., & Spittal, P. M. (2014b). Lost in transition: HIV Prevalence and correlates of infection among young people living in post-emergency phase transit camps in Gulu district, northern Uganda. *PLoS ONE, 9*(2), e89786. https://doi.org/10.1371/journal.pone.0089786

P'Bitek, O. 1971. *Religion of the central Luo.* East African Literature Bureau.

Pearshouse, R. (2014). An epidemic of bad laws: Building resistance. In L. Stackpool-Moore (Ed.), *HIV – Verdict on a virus: Public health, human rights and criminal law* (p. 14). https://www.ippf.org/sites/default/files/verdict_on_a_virus.pdf

Petersen, A., Davis, M., Fraser, S., & Lindsay, J. (2010). Healthy living and citizenship: An overview. *Critical Public Health, 20*(4), 391–400. https://doi.org/10.1080/09581596.2010.518379

Pfeiffer, J., & Nichter, M. (2008). What can critical medical anthropology contribute to global health? *Medical Anthropology Quarterly, 22*(4), 410–415. https://doi.org/10.1111/j.1548-1387.2008.00041.x

Pham, P. N., Vinck, P., & Stover, E. (2012). Abducted: The Lord's Resistance Army and forced conscription in Northern Uganda. *Human Rights Quarterly, 30*, 404–411. http://www.jstor.org/stable/20072848

Porter, H. E. (2012). Justice and rape on the periphery: The supremacy of social harmony in the space between local solutions and formal judicial systems in northern Uganda. *Journal of Eastern African Studies, 6*(1), 81–97. https://doi.org/10.1080/17531055.2012.664705

Ragoné, H. (1999). The gift of life. In L. Layne (Ed.), *Transformative motherhood: On giving and getting in a consumer culture.* New York University Press.

Rankin, J. M. (2015). The rhetoric of patient and family-centred care: An institutional ethnography into what actually happens. *Journal of Advanced Nursing, 71*(3), 526–534. https://doi.org/10.1111/jan.12575

Ray, A. M., & Salihu, H. M. (2004). The impact of maternal mortality interventions using traditional birth attendants and village midwives. *Journal of Obstetrics & Gynecology, 24*(1), 5–11. https://doi.org/10.1080/01443610310001620206

Rebick, J. (1993). Is the issue choice? In G. Basen, M. Eichler, & A. Lippmann (Eds.), *Misconceptions: The social construction of choice and the new reproductive technologies* (pp. 87–89). Voyageur Publishing.

Refugee Law Project. (2012). *Border or ownership question: The Apaa land dispute* [Briefing note]. http://www.refugeelawproject.org/resources/briefing-notes-special-reoprts/109-conflict-tj/sprpts-ctj-accs/270-border-or-ownership-question-the-apaa-land-dispute.html

Republic of Uganda. (2006). *Roadmap for reduction of maternal & neonatal mortality and morbidity.*

Republic of Uganda. (2014). *The HIV and AIDS Prevention and Control Act, 2014.* http://www.ilo.org/dyn/natlex/docs/ELECTRONIC/110805/137931/F-1081306421/UGA110805.pdf

Republic of Uganda. (2015). *Resettlement policy framework.* https://www.amuru.go.ug/publications/national-population-and-housing-census-2014-area-specific-profiles-amuru-district

Rieder, S. (2016). Interrogating the global health and development nexus: Critical viewpoints of neoliberalization and health in transnational spaces. *World Development Perspectives, 2,* 55–61. https://doi.org/10.1016/j.wdp.2016.10.004

Rogo, K. O., Oucho, J., & Mwalali, P. (2006). Maternal mortality. In D. T. Jamison, R. G. Feachem, M. W. Makgoba, E. R. Bos, F. K. Baingana, K. J. Hofman, & K. O. Rogo (Eds.), *Disease and mortality in sub-Saharan Africa* (2nd ed., pp. 223–236). The World Bank.

Rose, N. (2007). *The politics of life itself: Biomedicine, power, and subjectivity in the twenty-first century.* Princeton University Press.

Rossiter, K. (2012). Talking turkey: Anxiety, public health stories, and the responsibilization of health. *Journal of Canadian Studies/Revue d'études canadiennes, 46*(2), 178–195. https://www.muse.jhu.edu/article/515018

Rudrum, S. (2016a). Institutional ethnography research in global south settings: The role of texts. *International Journal of Qualitative Methods, 15*(1). https://doi.org/10.1177/1609406916637088

Rudrum, S. (2016b). Traditional birth attendants: Policy, practice, and ethics. *Healthcare for Women International, 37*(2), 250–269. https://doi.org/10.1080/07399332.2015.1020539

Rudrum, S. (2017). Pregnancy and birth in the global south: A review of critical approaches to sociocultural risk illustrated with fieldwork data from northern Uganda. *Health, Risk & Society, 19*(1–2), 1–18.

Rudrum, S., Brown, H., & Oliffe, J. L. (2016). Understanding the meaning and role of gifts given to Ugandan mothers in maternity care settings: "The help they give when they've seen how different you are." *Sociology of Health & Illness, 38*(8), 1318–1335. https://doi.org/10.1111/1467-9566.12456

Rudrum, S., Oliffe, J. L., & Brown, H. (2017). Antenatal care and couples' HIV testing in rural northern Uganda: A gender relations analysis. *American Journal of Men's Health, 11*(4), 811–822. https://doi.org/10.1177%2F1557988315602527

Ruhl, L. (1999). Liberal governance and prenatal care: Risk and regulation in pregnancy. *Economy and Society, 28*(1), 95–117. https://doi.org/10.1080/03085149900000026

Saith, A. (2006). From universal values to Millennium Development Goals: Lost in translation. *Development and Change, 37*(6), 1167–1199. https://doi.org/10.1111/j.1467-7660.2006.00518.x

Say, L., & Raine, R. (2007). A systematic review of inequalities in the use of maternal health care in developing countries: Examining the scale of the problem and the importance of context. *Bulletin of the World Health Organization, 85*, 812–819. https://doi.org/10.2471/blt.06.035659

Sebina-Zziwa, A., Nyamugasira, W., & Larok, A. (2013). *A long way to go: A civil society review of progress towards the Millennium Development Goals in Commonwealth countries.* Commonwealth Foundation.

Sen, A. (1999). *Commodities and capabilities.* Oxford University Press

Serwajja, E. (2018). The "green land grab" in Apaa village of Amuru district, northern Uganda: Power, complexities & consequences. *Mambo!, 15*(2). https://halshs.archives-ouvertes.fr/halshs-01734780/document

Sevigny, C. A. (2012). *Starting from refugees themselves: Sketch for an institutional ethnography of refugee resettlement* [Past winner of the CARFMS graduate student essay contest]. http://carfms.org/research-and-papers/carfms-student-essay-contest/graduate/

Shafer, L. A., Biraro, S., Nakiyingi-Miiro, J., Kamali, A., Ssematimba, D., Ouma, J., Ojiwiya, A., Hughes, P., Van der Paal, L., Whitworth, J., Opio, A., & Grosskurth, H. (2008). HIV prevalence and incidence are no longer falling in southwest Uganda: evidence from a rural population cohort 1989–2005. *AIDS, 22*(13), 1641–1649. https://doi.org/10.1097/QAD.0b013e32830a7502

Sia, D., Onadja, Y., Nandi, A., Foro, A., & Brewer, T. (2014). What lies behind Gender inequalities in HIV/AIDS in Sub-Saharan African countries: Evidence from Kenya, Lesotho and Tanzania. *Health Policy and Planning, 29*(7), 938–949. https://doi.org/10.1093/heapol/czt075

Sibley, L. M., Sipe, T. A., Brown, C. M., Diallo, M. M., McNatt, K., & Habarta, N. (2009). Traditional birth attendant training for improving health behaviours and pregnancy outcomes (Review). *The Cochrane Library, 2.*

Sinding, C. (2010). Using institutional ethnography to understand the production of health care disparities. *Qualitative Health Research, 20*(12), 1656–1663. https://doi.org/10.1177/1049732310377452

Smith, D. E. (1987). *The everyday world as problematic: A feminist sociology.* University of Toronto Press.

Smith, D. E. (1990). *Texts, facts, and femininity: Exploring the relations of ruling.* Routledge.

Smith, D. E. (1997). From the margins: Women's standpoint as a method of inquiry in the social sciences. *Gender,* Technology and Development, *1*(1), 113–135. https://doi.org/10.1177/097185249700100106

Smith, D. E. (2002). *Texts, facts and femininity: Exploring the relations of ruling.* Routledge.

Smith, D. E. (2005). *Institutional ethnography: A sociology for people.* Rowman Altamira.

Smith, D. E. (Ed.). (2006). *Institutional ethnography as practice.* Rowman & Littlefield.

Smith, D. E. (2014). Discourse as social relations: Sociological theory and the dialogic of sociology. In D. E. Smith & S. M. Turner (Eds.), *Incorporating texts into institutional ethnographies* (pp. 225–251). University of Toronto Press.

Smith, L. T. (1999). *Decolonizing methodologies: Research and Indigenous peoples.* Zed Books.

Spangler, S. A. (2011). "To open oneself is a poor woman's trouble": Embodied inequality and childbirth in south-central Tanzania. *Medical Anthropology Quarterly, 25*(4), 479–498. https://doi.org/10.1111/j.1548-1387.2011.01181.x

Spittal, P., Muyinda, H., Oyat, G., & Patel, S. (2008). *The Wayo programme: Building on child and traditional assets in supporting Acholi young women and girls in the context of HIV, war and post conflict.* CIDA Child Protection Fund

Ssengooba, F., Neema, S., Mbonye, A., Sentubwe, O., & Onama, V. (2003). *Maternal health review Uganda.* https://assets.publishing.service.gov.uk/media/57a08d20ed915d3cfd001826/04-03_uganda.pdf

Stewart, B. (2012, December 15). A missing perspective: Children born into LRA captivity. *The Sky Is Yellow.* http://theskyisyellownow.blogspot.ca/2012/03/missing-perspective-children-born-into.html

Stirrat, R. L., & Henkel, H. (1997). The development gift: The problem of reciprocity in the NGO world. *The Annals of the American Academy of Political and Social Science, 554*(1), 66–80. https://doi.org/10.1177%2F0002716297554001005

Sundby, J. (2014). A rollercoaster of policy shifts: Global trends and reproductive health policy in the Gambia. *Global Public Health, 9*(8), 894–909. https://doi.org/10.1080/17441692.2014.940991

Taylor, J. J. (2007). Assisting or compromising intervention? The concept of "culture" in biomedical and social research on HIV/AIDS. *Social Science & Medicine, 64*(4), 965–975.

Tegulle, G. (2013). Why traditional birth attendants will keep thriving. *The Monitor.* Retrieved January 15, 2014, from http://www.monitor.co.ug/artsculture/Reviews/Why-traditional-birth-attendants-will-keep-thriving/-/691232/1845284/-/12o3ca8z/-/index.html

Thompson, L., & Kumar, A. (2011). Responses to health promotion campaigns: resistance, denial and othering. *Critical Public Health, 21*(1), 105–117. https://doi.org/10.1080/09581591003797129

Titmuss, R. (1970). *The gift relationship.* The New Press.

Trostle, J. A. (1988). Medical compliance as an ideology. *Social Science & Medicine, 27*(12), 1299–1308. https://doi.org/10.1016/0277-9536(88)90194-3

Turinawe, E. B., Rwemisisi, J. T., Musinguzi, L. K., de Groot, M., Muhangi, D., de Vries, D. H., Mafigiri, D. K., Katamba, A., Parker, N., & Pool, R. (2016). Traditional birth attendants (TBAs) as potential agents in promoting male involvement in maternity preparedness: insights from a rural community in Uganda. *Reproductive Health, 13*(24), 1–11, https://doi.org/10.1186/s12978-016-0147-7

Uganda Bureau of Statistics. (2011). *Uganda demographic and health survey.*

Uganda Bureau of Statistics. (2016). *Uganda demographic and health survey.*

Uganda Ministry of Health. (2006). *Roadmap for accelerating the reduction of maternal and neonatal mortality and morbidity in Uganda, 2007–2015.* https://www.who.int/pmnch/media/events/2013/uganda_mnh_roadmap.pdf

Uganda Ministry of Health. (2010). *VHT strategy and operational guidelines.*

Uganda Ministry of Health. (2016). *Uganda clinical guidelines: National guidelines for management of common conditions.* http://library.health.go.ug/download/file/fid/429

*Uganda: Land disputes threaten northern peace.* (2012). IRIN News. http://www.irinnews.org/report/95322/uganda-land-disputes-threaten-northern-peace

Uganda Ministry of Finance, Planning and Economic Development. (2013). *Millennium Development Goals port for Uganda, 2013.* https://www.undp.org/content/dam/uganda/docs/UNDPUg-2013MDGProgress%20Report-Oct%202013.pdf

United Nations Population Fund. (2014). *Skilled attendance at birth.* http://
www.unfpa.org/public/mothers/pid/4383

United States Agency for International Development. (2015). *Uganda's private
health sector: Opportunities for growth.* https://banyanglobal.com/wp-content
/uploads/2017/07/Ugandas-Private-Health-Sector-Opportunities-for
-Growth.pdf

Vallières, F., Hansen, A., McAuliffe, E., Cassidy, E. L., Owora, P., Kappler, S., &
Gathuru, E. (2013). Head of household education level as a factor influencing
whether delivery takes place in the presence of a skilled birth attendant in
Busia, Uganda: A cross-sectional household study. *BMC Pregnancy and
Childbirth, 13*(48), 1–8. https://doi.org/10.1186/1471-2393-13-48

Van Lerberghe, W., & De Brouwere, V. (2000). Reducing maternal mortality
in a context of poverty. *Safe motherhood strategies: A review of the evidence*
(Vol. 17). ITG Press.

Venkatapuram, S., Bell, R., & Marmot, M. (2010). The right to sutures: Social
epidemiology, human rights, and social justice. *Health and Human Rights,
12*(2), 3–16. https://www.ncbi.nlm.nih.gov/pmc/articles/PMC3694312/

Vernooij, E., & Hardon, A. (2013). "What mother wouldn't want to save her
baby?" HIV testing and counselling practices in a rural Ugandan antenatal
clinic. *Culture, Health & Sexuality, 15*(S4), S553–S566. https://doi.org
/10.1080/13691058.2012.758314

Walker, N., Stanecki, K. A., Brown, T., Stover, J., Lazzari, S., Garcia-Calleja,
J. M., Schwartländer, B., & Ghys, P. D. (2003). Methods and procedures
for estimating HIV/AIDS and its impact: the UNAIDS/WHO estimates
for the end of 2001. *AIDS, 17*(15), 2215–2225. https://doi.org/10.1097/01
.aids.0000076339.42412.2b

Wawer, M. J., Makumbi, F., Kigozi, G., Serwadda, D., Watya, S., Nalugoda, F.,
Buwembo, D., Ssempijja, V., Kiwanuka, N., Moulton, L. H., Sewankambo,
N. K., Reynolds, S. J., Quinn, T. C., Opendi, P., Iga, B., Ridzon, R.,
Laeyendecker, O., & Gray, R. H. (2009). Circumcision in HIV-infected men
and its effect on HIV transmission to female partners in Rakai, Uganda:
A randomised controlled trial. *The Lancet, 374*(9685), 229–237. https://doi
.org/10.1016/S0140-6736(09)60998-3

Webb, M. (2012, February 16). Uganda nature reserve dispute turns deadly.
*Al Jazeera.* https://www.aljazeera.com/video/africa/2012/02
/2012216114011916292.html

Weber, L. (2006). Reconstructing the landscape of health disparities research:
promoting dialogue and collaboration between feminist intersectional
and biomedical paradigms. In A. Schulz & L. Mullings (Eds.), *Race, Class,
Gender and Health* (pp. 21–59). Jossey-Bass.

Westerhaus, M. (2007). Linking anthropological analysis and epidemiological
evidence: Formulating a narrative of HIV transmission in Acholiland of

northern Uganda. *SAHARA-J: Journal of Social Aspects of HIV/AIDS, 4*(2), 590–605. https://doi.org/10.1080/17290376.2007.9724881

Westerhaus, M. J., Finnegan, A. C., Zabulon, Y., & Mukherjee, J. S. (2007). Framing HIV prevention discourse to encompass the complexities of war in northern Uganda. *American Journal of Public Health, 97*(7), 1184–1186. https://doi.org/10.2105/AJPH.2005.072777

Whyte, S. R., Whyte, M. A., Meinert, L., & Twebaze, J. (2013). Therapeutic clientship. In J. Biehl & A. Petryna (Eds.), *When people come first* (pp. 140–165). Princeton University Press.

Wilkinson, S. (1998). Focus groups in health research exploring the meanings of health and illness. *Journal of Health Psychology, 3*(3), 329–348. https://doi .org/10.1177/135910539800300304

Wilson, A., Lissauer, D., Thangaratinam, S., Khan, K. S., MacArthur, C., & Coomarasamy, A. (2011). A comparison of clinical officers with medical doctors on outcomes of caesarean section in the developing world: Meta-analysis of controlled studies. *BMJ: British Medical Journal, 342*, 1–8. https:// doi.org/10.1136/bmj.d2600

Wirth, M., Sacks, E., Delamonica, E., Storeygard, A., Minujin, A., & Balk, D. (2008). "Delivering" on the MDGs?: Equity and maternal health in Ghana, Ethiopia and Kenya. *East African Journal of Public Health, 5*(3), 133–141. https://www.ncbi.nlm.nih.gov/pmc/articles/PMC4414036/

Women Deliver. (2009). *Focus on 5: Women's health and the MDGs.* https://www .unfpa.org/sites/default/files/pub-pdf/Focus-on-5.pdf

Women of Uganda Network. (2013, June 11). *Five health workers of Otwee Health Centre III in Amuru Town arrested over negligent of duty.* https://ict4dem.blogs .dsv.su.se/five-health-workers-of-otwee-health-centre-iii-in-amuru-town -council-arrested-over-negligence-of-duty/

World Health Organization. (n.d.). *Millennium Development Goal 5.* http://www .who.int/reproductivehealth/topics/mdgs/target_5a/en/

World Health Organization. (1992). *Traditional birth attendants: A joint WHO/ UNFPA/UNICEF statement.*

World Health Organization. (2004). *Making pregnancy safer: The critical role of the skilled attendant. A joint statement by WHO, ICM and FIGO.* https://www .who.int/maternal_child_adolescent/documents/9241591692/en/

World Health Organization. (2012). *End of Ebola outbreak in Uganda.* https:// www.who.int/csr/don/2012_10_04/en/

World Health Organization. (2014). *Skilled attendance.*

World Health Organization. (2016). *New guidelines on antenatal care for a positive pregnancy experience.* https://www.who.int/reproductivehealth/news /antenatal-care/en/

Yamin, A. E. (2013). From ideals to tools: Applying human rights to maternal health. *PLoS Medicine, 10*(11), e1001546. https://doi.org/10.1371/journal .pmed.1001546

Yamin, A. E., & Boulanger, V. M. (2013). Embedding sexual and reproductive health and rights in a transformational development framework: Lessons learned from the MDG targets and indicators. *Reproductive Health Matters, 21*(42), 74–85. https://doi.org/10.1016/S0968-8080(13)42727-1

Young, I. M. (2008). Structural injustice and the politics of difference. In E. Grabham, D. Cooper, J. Krishnadas, & D. Herman (Eds.), *Intersectionality and beyond: Law, power and the politics of location* (pp. 273–298). Routledge-Cavendish

Zaba, B., Boerma, T., & White, R. (2000). Monitoring the AIDS epidemic using HIV prevalence data among young women attending antenatal clinics: Prospects and problems. *AIDS, 14*(11), 1633–1645. https://doi.org/10.1097/00002030-200007280-00020

Zarowsky, C. (2000). Poverty, pity, and the erasure of power: Somali refugee dependency. In L. M. Whiteford & L. Manderson (Eds.), *Global health policy, local realities: The fallacy of the level playing field* (pp. 177–204). Lynne Reinner Publishers.

Zola, I. K. (1981). Structural constraints in the doctor-patient relationship: the case of non-compliance. In L. Eisenberg & A. Kleinman. (Eds.), *The relevance of social science for medicine* (pp. 241–252). Reidel.

# Index

www.ingramcontent.com/pod-product-compliance
Lightning Source LLC
LaVergne TN
LVHW092006221224
799610LV00011B/105/J